RAW PT, v.4.0

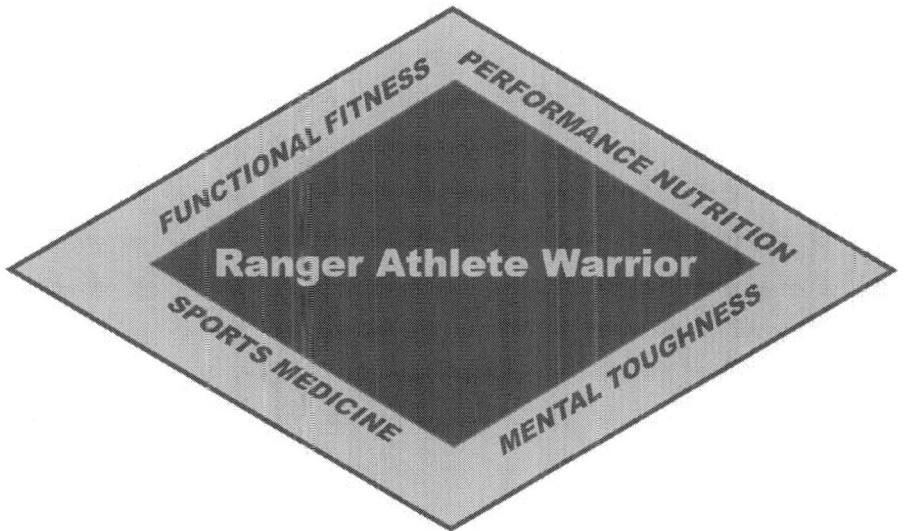

Further, Faster, Harder

Table of Contents

__PURPOSE OF RAW__ is to provide education and training that optimize the physical/mental development and sustainment of the Regiment's most lethal weapon - the individual Ranger.

The __END-STATE OBJECTIVE OF RAW__ is to field self-sustaining systems that ensure all Rangers:

> Achieve a level of physical fitness that is commensurate with the physical requirements of Ranger missions.

> Understand and choose sound nutritional practices.

> Employ mental toughness skills to enhance personal and professional development.

> Receive screening/education for injury prevention and prompt, effective, and thorough treatment/rehabilitation of injuries when they do occur.

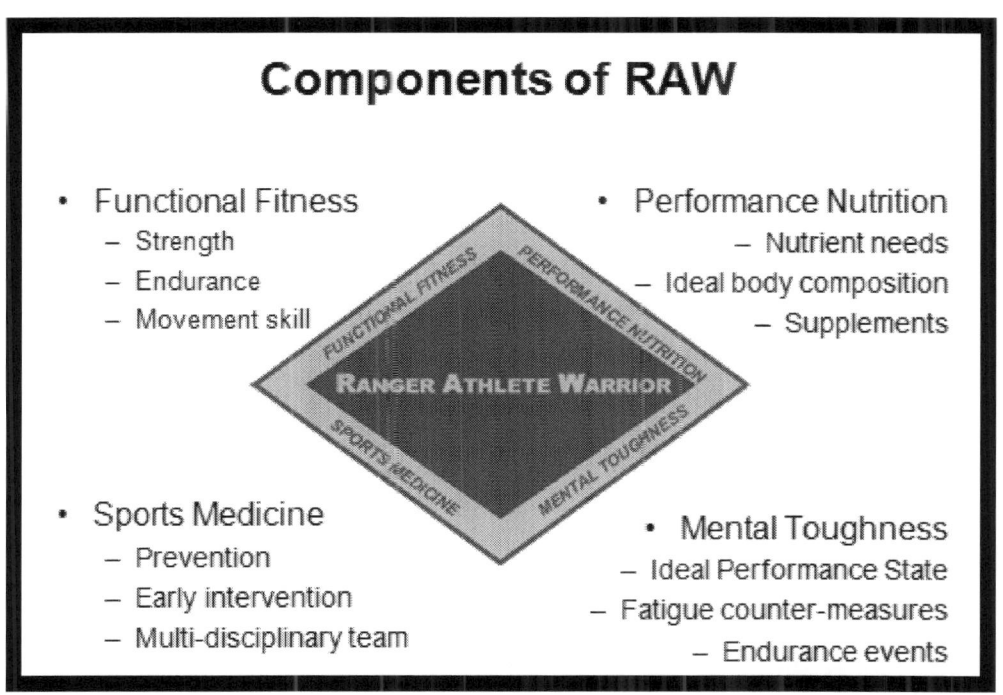

RAW Philosophy

- The individual Ranger is the Regiment's most lethal weapon.

- You don't know how tough your next enemy will be. Assume he'll be very tough.

- You don't know exactly what the physical requirement will be on your next mission. Assume it will be extremely demanding.

- Ranger missions require strength, endurance, and movement skills…excelling in only one or two leaves you vulnerable to poor performance and/or injuries.

- Training hard is not enough; you have to train smart as well.

- As an individual, a team, a squad, or a platoon, you are only as strong as your weakest link. Don't have a weak link.

- Form matters. Master the exercise techniques and demand proper execution from your men.

- The body adapts to the stress you place upon it. This takes time. Cells aren't necessarily on the same schedule as your head and your heart. In other words, be consistent, patient, and think of improvement over weeks and months, not days.

- Don't crush yourself everyday. Respect the need for recovery. RAW scheduling guidance builds in some degree of recovery, but leaders must be attuned to their men and modify the training stress appropriately.

- Fuel the machine. Don't train well then blow it with a lousy diet. Have a plan for hydration and meals/snacks and stick to it.

- Take care of your injuries before they become chronic. Playing hurt is necessary on occasion, but do it too long and there may not be a therapy or surgery fix.

- Keep your head in the game. Historically, warriors have been defined more by their minds than their bodies. Similarly, most athletes claim their performance is as much mental as physical, yet they seldom train or have a plan for developing mental toughness. Rangers need to recognize their ideal performance state and be able to call it up at a moment's notice.

- Learn all you can about your mind, your body, nutrition, and exercise, and then apply that to the task at hand…making you and your Rangers the best tactical athletes on the planet.

- Bottom Line: Train right, eat right, sleep right, and keep your head in the game.

Principles of Exercise

- Progression: Following this principle means that you take a systematic approach to increasing the physical demands over time. For example, if your squad has been performing long runs of 35 minutes and you want to progress to 60, then you need a plan for doing so. The general rule-of-thumb is to progress time/distance by no more than 10% per week. When you do the math, you see that it will take about six weeks to safely progress from 35 to 60 minutes. The principle of gradual progression is just as important for resistance training. Start by mastering core stability and control of body-weight exercises. Add external resistance and/or volume (number of reps over a given period of time) gradually as long as control of the movement is well-maintained. Many injuries can be traced to attempting workouts that are beyond an individual's current capability.

- Regularity: This one is pretty obvious. Rangers don't generally have a problem with this. However, two points should be noted. First, if for whatever reason you cannot do PT for two or more consecutive weeks, assume you've lost some degree of fitness. You should then resume PT at a lower level and gradually build back up. Second, even though you may be doing PT on a regular basis, if you stop doing a particular component of PT (agility or plyometric training, for example), then you should re-master the basics of those drills before jumping back into an aggressive workout. Note that endurance is lost faster than strength.

- Overload: To improve strength, endurance, or movement skills, you must provide a stimulus. This means moving outside your comfort zone…progressively lifting a little more, running a little faster or farther, practicing agility drills that don't come easy, etc. It is extremely easy to overload. The challenge is to do it intelligently. You must apply the principles of progression and recovery together with overload.

- Variety: Over the years, researchers and trainers have learned that athletes maximize their potential by dedicating a given period of time to a particular aspect of physical development, then changing the focus at regular intervals. For example, many strength programs begin with the focus on mass-producing workouts, then strength, later emphasizing general power training, and finally move to activity-specific strength/power drills. Such regular changes to workouts force the body to continue adapting. If you stay with the same routine, the body becomes accustomed to it and development stops. Maintaining variety in a program also helps to control overuse injuries. If all of your endurance training comes from running, you are more susceptible to stress-related injuries (stress fracture, tendinitis, etc.). Finally, variety in physical training is absolutely necessary to be prepared for the broad-ranging physical requirements of Ranger missions.

- Recovery: The principle of recovery is closely related to the principles of overload and progression. Overload must be followed by some degree of recovery. Some workouts demand more recovery than others. Sessions that aggressively train speed, power, jumping/landing/cutting or heavy lifting should be followed by either a day of rest or PT than involves a moderate session of some other component (an easy run/swim and some mat-based core training, for example). Regarding progression and recovery, some periods, whether it is a day, a week, or several weeks, will involve PT that is relatively easy compared to the hardest days or training cycles. Another way of saying this is: you should not be red-lining every day nor burned out at the end of each week. Attempting to maintain maximal workouts for several months runs the risk of overtraining, which is related to not only muscles/bones/tendons stress injuries, but also disruption of hormonal balance. By incorporating relatively less training intensity and volume during a portion of the training cycle, the body is much less likely to breakdown.

- Balance: For Rangers, a balanced approach to PT scheduling means your program consistently incorporates training that develops strength, endurance, and movement skills (power, agility, coordination, etc). Taking this notion a step further, strength must be balanced by performing some workouts with body-weight resistance, some with moderate-heavy resistance, and some with a moderate resistance that is moved quickly (power training). Endurance should be balanced by performing a mix of aerobic and anaerobic training.

- Specificity: Following this principle ensures that you will be fit for the important stuff. Whenever the idea of fitness is discussed, the question "Fit for what?" should be part of the discussion. For Rangers, the answer is "Fit for current and potential Ranger training and combat missions." This doesn't mean that every workout must look like a combat mission. It does mean that you should always be aware of your big-picture PT objectives and understand how each workout, each week, each month of PT contribute to it. At least part of a training cycle needs to focus directly on tactical fitness. Such training must involve an operationally relevant degree of intensity and volume, but should be preceded by general fitness development (strength, endurance, movement skills).

- Precision: This term refers to the biomechanical correctness of movement. We know through observation and research that some movement patterns are efficient and effective, while other are inefficient and possibly destructive (over time, likely to lead to injury). For example, spinal stability not only protects the spine but also creates a stable base of support from which the arms and legs can generate power. Rangers should study and master optimal execution for all drills in the program. There will be times during training when we must push ourselves through fatigue and perhaps sacrifice perfect form. However, these should be the exceptions and not the everyday norms.

Understanding Movement Prep and Recovery

Movement preparation and recovery are vital pieces of the RAW PT program. In the past, they've been known as warm-up and cool-down. In keeping with the terms used by most top trainers, the names have been change to reflect the intent of the drills.

Movement preparation is a better term than warm-up. Preparing the body to move well is precisely the goal. Warming the body is part of movement prep, but it is no more important than the other two objectives of movement prep: loosening the joints/muscles, and priming the nerve to muscle messages. If warming were the only objective, you could sit in a sauna and call it warm-up. After movement prep, Rangers should be prepared to run, lift, negotiate obstacles, play a sport, and execute a raid...

The movement prep recommended for Rangers is very similar to that used by top strength and conditioning coaches. It is somewhat different than the 5-step warm-up described in the Army's Physical Fitness Training FM (circa 1980s). While that warm-up was based on sound principles at the time, in the past decade research has shown that static stretching during warm-up is not necessary for injury prevention or performance.

The term recovery is used instead of cool-down. Similar to the idea of warm-up as only a component of movement prep, cooling down is only a small part of recovery. The objectives of recovery are 1) safely decrease heart-rate, respiratory rate, and body temperature, 2) improve functional flexibility; 3) replace nutrients, and 4) rest enough so that the body is ready for subsequent PT or missions.

Only the first two objectives are met on the PT field. This means that meeting objectives three and four are a personal responsibility. Leaders must educate and motivate their men to follow the nutritional and sleep guidelines put forth in the RAW classes.

It is clear that many individuals blow off cool-down and go straight to the shower without any obvious ill effects. Leaders should discourage this practice. Performing the functional flexibility exercises in the recovery drill will identify areas of tightness that might eventually lead to injury or limit performance. Those exercises were in fact designed to do just that. Obviously not everyone will need every stretch. However, those Rangers that do find areas of tightness or restriction during recovery stretches should be encouraged to repeat the stretches throughout the day.

Performing an organized recovery session offers squad leaders at least two other benefits: 1) the opportunity to provide the men with immediate feedback on the performance of the PT session, and 2) the opportunity to remind the men to re-hydrate and get the proper nutrients at the proper time.

To enhance recovery after PT, alternating heat and cold treatments may be of value. The easiest way to accomplish this is in the shower after PT. Another recovery enhancer that many Rangers find useful is the foam roll. Think of these tools as self-massage aids. See the battalion HPOC or PT for further guidance on recovery practices.

Movement Prep

Purpose: Bring metabolism from rest to exercise levels, loosen the major joints and muscle groups, prime nerve-to-muscle messages that improve total-body coordination – all in preparation for any physical activity that follows.

Utilization: Before each PT session in all phases. Movement prep should be completed in about 10 minutes.

Execution: Calisthenics may be performed in an extended, rectangular formation for large groups or in a circle for squads. Perform 3-5 repetitions for each exercise, beginning with slow movements through an easy range-of-motion, adding just a little speed and range-of motion with each repetition. Perform the movement drills as indicate below, using an extended, rectangular formation. The last four movement drills are performed over a 20 meter distance. Pause as need between exercises to avoid fatigue. After movement prep, the body should be warm, loose and primed for intense activity – but not fatigued.

Calisthenics	Movement Drills
Bend and Reach	Side-Step Lunge (5 reps then reverse).
Around the World	Corkscrew Lunge (5 reps then reverse)
Squat	Walking Lunge & Reach (10 steps each leg)
Windmill	Walking Bend and Reach (10 steps each leg)
Leg Whips	Verticals (down and back)
Balance and Reach, Rearward	Laterals (down and back)
Pushup+/Pushups/Rotations	Crossovers (down and back)
Squat-Reach-Jump	Shuttle Run (down-back-down)

Bend and Reach

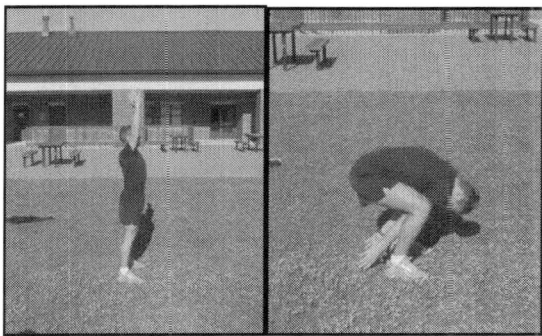

- Start and finish with the arms overhead, abs engaged; don't lean backward.
- At the bottom of the movement, knees are bent, back round, head down looking and reaching between legs.
- Perform at a slow cadence.
- Perform 3-5 repetitions.

Squat

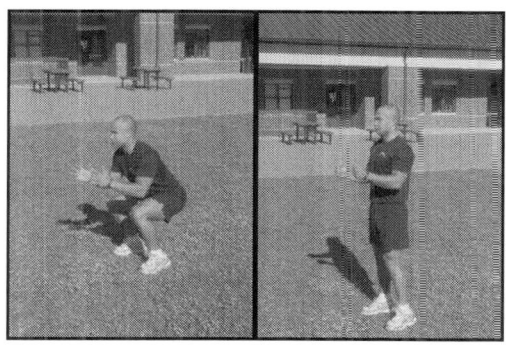

- Start and end with the arms in the ready position.
- Squat so that the knees are aligned over the toes, heels are down, the back is straight, the head and chest are up.
- Perform 3-5 repetitions.

Around the World

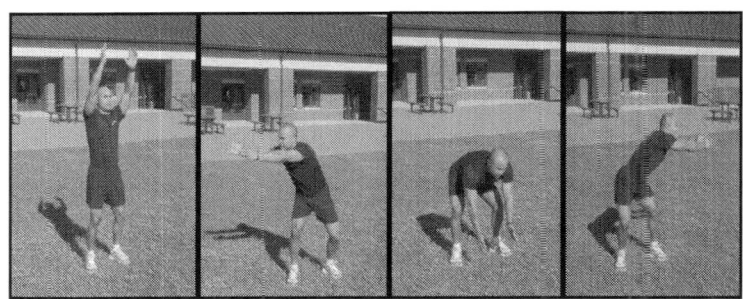

- Start and finish with the arms overhead, abs engaged.
- Perform slow, continuous, circular movements, especially stretching the side of the trunk.
- Perform clockwise and counterclockwise.
- Perform 3-5 repetitions.

Windmill

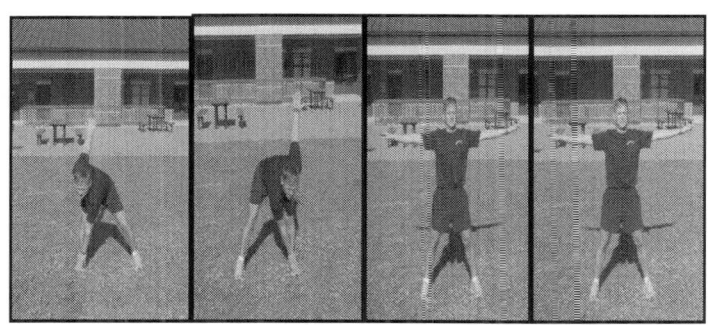

- Start in a wide stance with the arms to the side at shoulder level.
- Begin to squat, then rotate the hips and trunk to reach toward the opposite foot.
- Stay balanced, with slightly more weight on the side of the reach.
- Keep the head and chest relatively up.
- Perform 3-5 repetitions.

Leg Whips

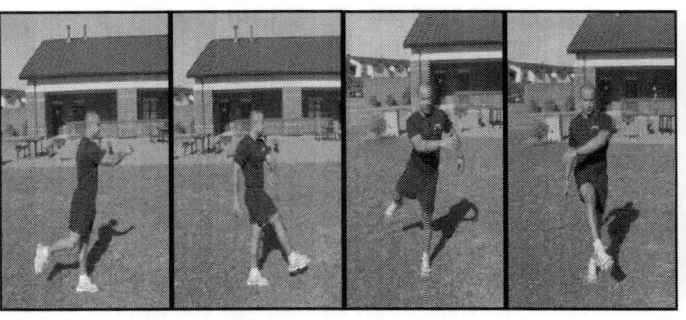

- Start and finish with the arms overhead, abs engaged.
- Perform slow, continuous, circular movements, especially stretching the side of the trunk.
- Perform clockwise and counterclockwise.
- Perform 3-5 repetitions.

Pushup +/Pushups/Rotations

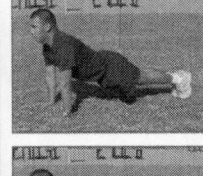
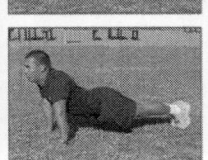
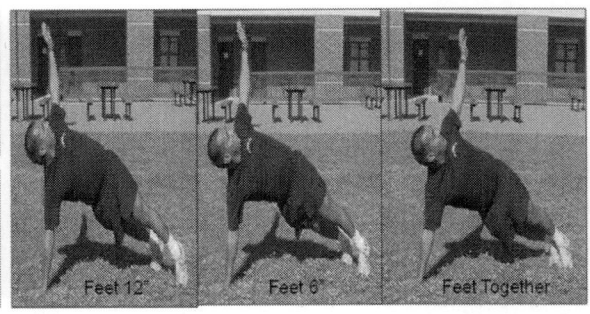

- Start in the pushup position with the elbows straight, with the movement occurring through the shoulder blades.
- Perform 10 pushups.
- From the top of the PU+ position, raise the left hand toward the sky, pause for one second, then return to the starting position and switch sides. Feet are 12" apart on first rep, 6" on second rep, together 3rd rep.
- Keep the trunk straight and abs tight throughout.
- Perform 3-5 repetitions.

Balance and Reach

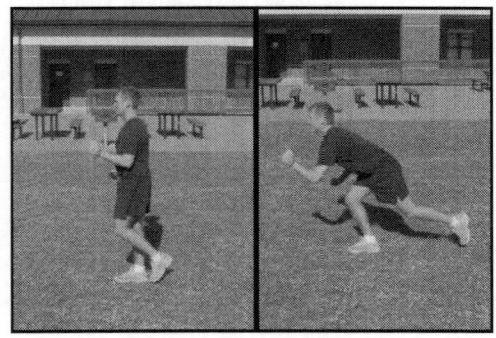

- From a single-leg stance, reach back with the other leg while counter-balancing with a forward lean of the trunk.
- The stance knee remains centered over the ball of the foot; do not let the knee waiver side-to-side.
- If the left leg is reaching back, the left arm is reaching forward.
- Perform 3-5 repetitions.

Squat-Reach-Jump

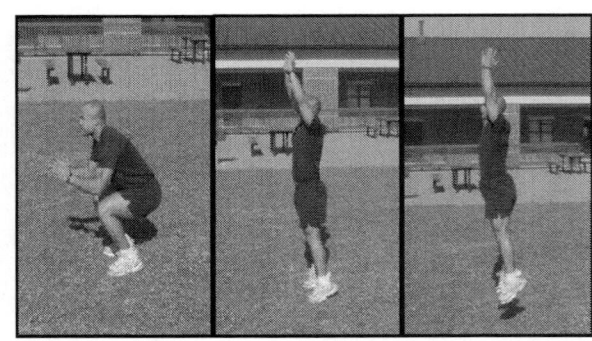

- Perform 5 squats as per the guidance for the squat exercise
- Perform 5 reaches by rising out of the squat onto the toes and reaching overhead
- Perform 5 jumps. Landings should be soft (balls of the feet first, then sinking to heels), with impact absorbed by plenty of bend of the hips and knees. Keep the feet shoulder width apart or less. Do not allow the knees to buckle inward or outward upon landing.
- Perform 3-5 repetitions.

Side Step Lunge

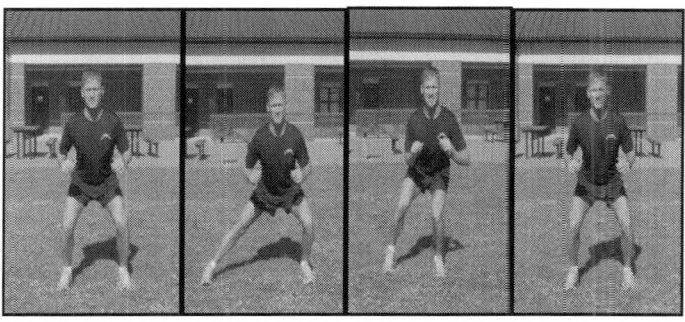

- Squat first, then stay in the crouch and step to the side. A slight stretch should be felt in the groin as the trail leg straightens.
- Stay in the crouch with the trunk upright and bring the trail leg back to the squat position.
- After 5 side-steps, stand up to recover for a couple seconds, then repeat in the opposite direction.

Corkscrew Lunge

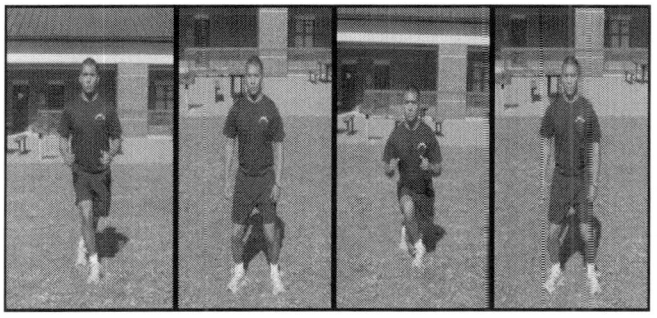

- Step to the rear with the trail leg, crossing it behind the forward leg.
- Leaving the legs in place, rotate the trunk back to the front (3rd picture), as you sink into a squat. A stretch will be felt in the glutes of the forward leg.
- Return to the starting position by pushing off the front leg. Perform 5 repetitions on each side.

Walking Lunge and Reach

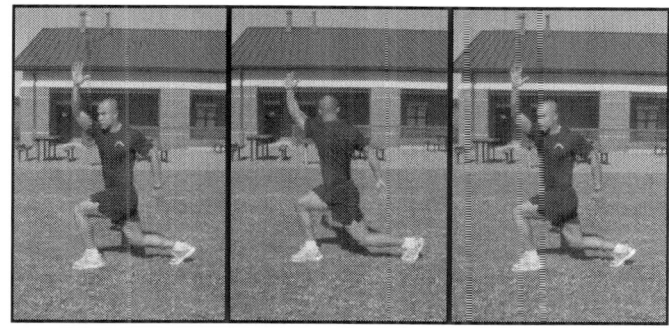

- Perform a full forward lunge, keeping the trunk upright and the abs tight.
- Rotate the trunk toward the side of the forward leg and sink into the lunge position. A stretch should be felt in the hip flexors of the rear leg. Pause in this position for just 1-2 seconds.
- Rise out of the lunge using the power of the front leg, then step through to perform the exercise on the opposite side. Perform 5 lunges with each leg.

Walking Bend and Reach

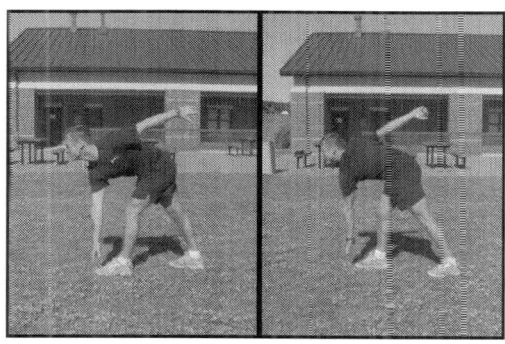

- Step forward with the leg while bending forward at the waist.
- Keep the trunk as straight as possible while reaching toward the opposite foot. A gentle stretch should be felt in the hamstring of the forward leg.
- Rise slowly out of the stretch, then step through to perform the exercise on the opposite side. Perform 5 reps with each leg.

Verticals

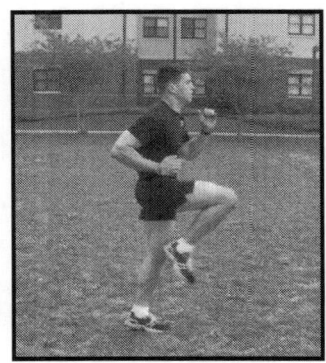

- Also known as the high-knee drill. Take short, quick strides, stay on the balls of the feet. The knees rise to waist level.
- Use strong arm action. The elbows stay bent at 90 degrees and reach well to the rear during the backswing. The hand of the forward arm moves to about chin level.
- Keep the trunk perpendicular to the ground.
- Perform over 20 yards, down and back.

Crossovers

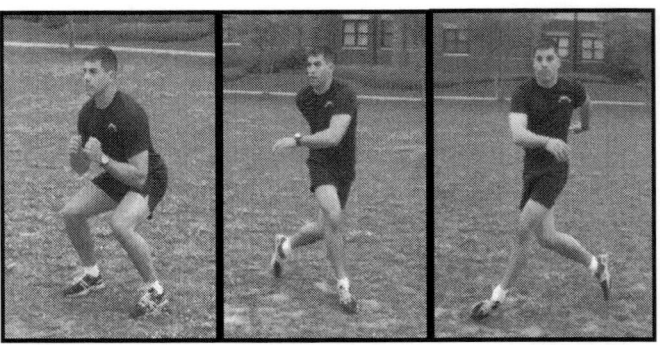

- Same starting position as laterals, but move laterally with crossover steps. The trail leg crosses first to the front, then to the rear
- The arms stay in the ready position or move counter to the leg crossover.
- Let the hips swivel rather than holding the trunk and pelvis stiffly.
- Perform 20 yards in each direction.

Laterals

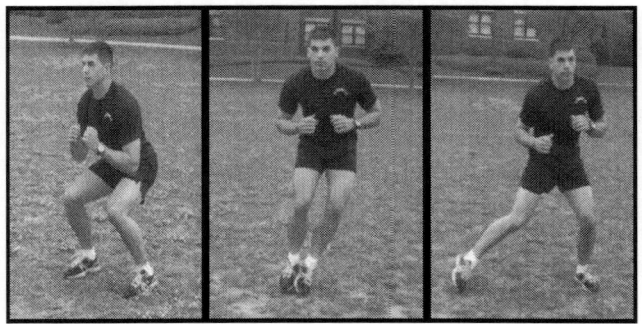

- Start in the power stance crouch, on the balls of the feet. Move laterally with shuffle steps
- Keep the feet directed to the front.
- Keep the back straight, the shoulder blades pulled slightly to the rear, and the hands in the ready position.
- Perform 20 yards in each direction.

Shuttle Run

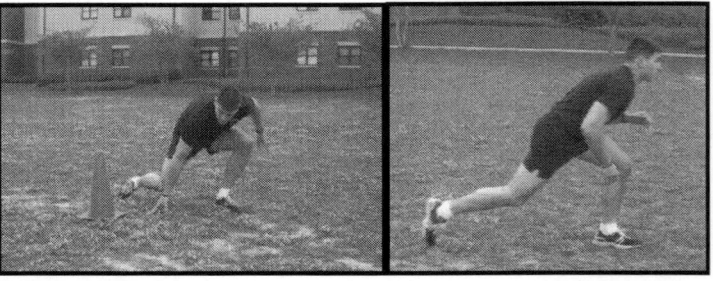

- Run at a moderate pace to the 20yard line and back, staying with the squad leader, then on the last 20yard segment, release into an 80% effort sprint.
- Always turn in the direction of the squad leader by making a half turn and crouching at the line, taking care to stay balanced and avoid twisting of the knees and ankle.

Recovery Flexibility Drill

Purpose: Safely decrease heart-rate, respiratory rate, body temperature; improve functional flexibility; replace nutrients.

Utilization: After each PT session in all phases

Execution: Walk as needed to bring the heart rate back to within about 20-30 beats of the resting level, then finish with the exercises below. The exercises with an * are considered motion exercises rather than static stretches, and need only be held for 1-3 seconds, 3-4 reps each side. The other exercises are stretches and should be held for 15-30s, 1 rep. The last four stretches are performed in standing. Rangers that find tight muscle groups should be encouraged to stretch on their own throughout the day. The stretch routine also provides a good opportunity for squad leaders to give their men feedback on the PT session.

Immediately after the PT session, re-hydrate and restore nutrients. The optimal post-exercise meal for the RAW program meets the following criteria: 1) ingested within 30 minutes, 2) about 3:1 ratio of carbs to protein, 3) at least 250 calories.

Exercise Order:

Mountain Climber Stretch
Seated Hip Rotations*
Quadriceps Stretch (side-lying)
Posterior Hip Stretch (supine)
Scorpion*
Rotational Spine Stretch (supine)*
Prone Press*
Prayer Stretch w/Diagonals
Hip Flexor Stretch
Hamstring Stretch
2-Part Gastroc-Soleus Stretch (wall or partner)
Pectoralis Stretch (wall or partner)

Mountain Climber Stretch

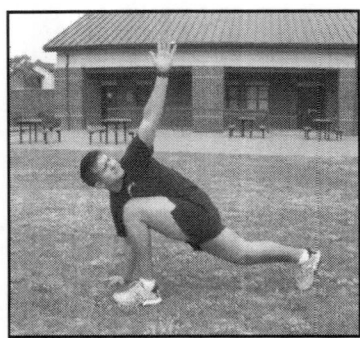

- Assume the starting position for the mountain climber exercise, except the forward foot is flat and the rearward leg fully extended.
- Keep the thigh of the forward leg tucked tightly into the trunk, then lift the arm on that side toward the sky, turning the trunk and head to look up.
- Hold for at least 15 seconds.

Quadriceps Stretch

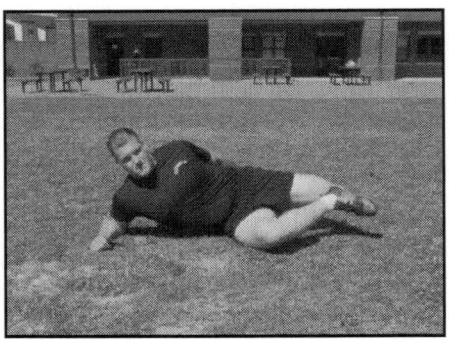

- Pull the thigh to the rear without straining the knee joint.
- Keep the abs tight to prevent the trunk from arching.
- Keep upper thigh parallel to the ground (or lower) as you stretch it.
- The lower leg can be used to nudge the stretch leg farther to the rear.
- Hold for at least 15 seconds.

Seated Hip Rotations

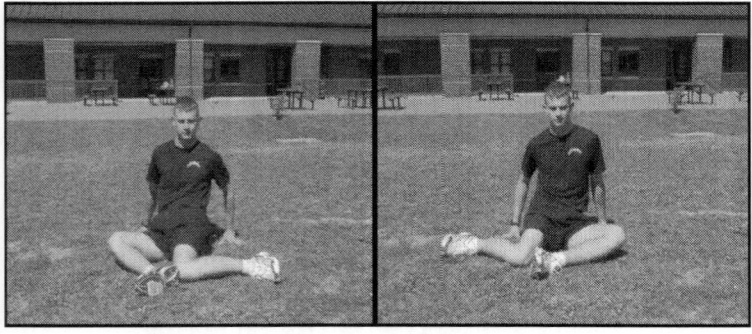

- From the position shown above, rotate the legs side to side.
- Keep the glutes and heels in place throughout the exercise.
- The trunk should face slightly away from the direction of the knees.
- If form is good and the exercise is painless, advance to hands in the ready position or overhead.
- Perform slow movements from side to side rather than holding as a static stretch.

Posterior Hip Stretch

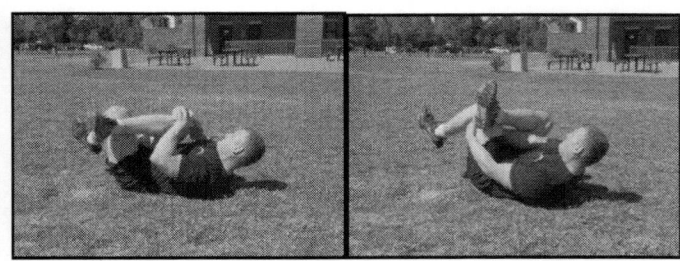

- Cross the ankle over the opposite knee and reach between the legs to pull both toward the chest. A stretch should be felt in the glutes of the crossed leg.
- An alternate method (picture on the right), is to cross the ankle over the knee, then pull the knee of the crossed leg toward the opposite shoulder.
- For both versions, the non-stretch leg should exert slight pressure pushing the crossed leg toward the chest.
- Hold for at least 15 seconds.

Scorpion

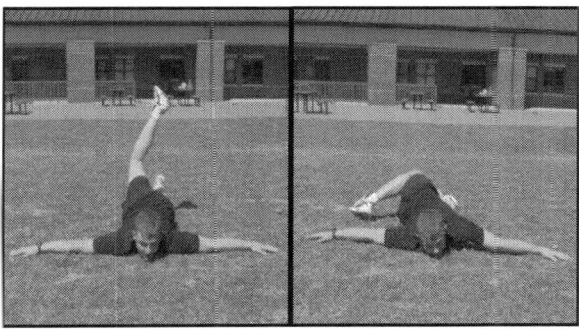

- Start in the prone position with the arms at the "T" position.
- Bend the left knee to 90 degrees, then lift the leg a few inches.
- Keeping the arms on the ground, slowly rotate the trunk to move the heel toward the opposite hand.
- Perform slow movements from side to side rather than holding as a stretching
- Perform 3-5 repetitions.

Prone Press

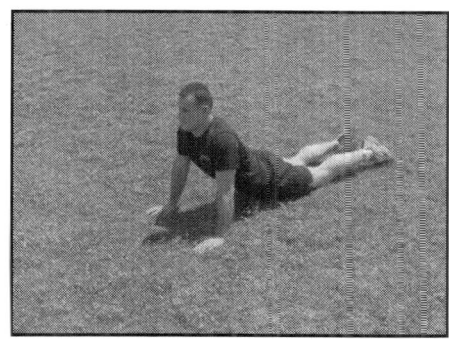

- From the prone position, press up leaving the legs, pelvis, and lower abdomen on the ground.
- Perform slow movement to the end range and pause briefly, rather than holding as a traditional static stretch.
- This exercise alternates with the Prayer Stretch. Perform three reps of each.
- Hold for 10 seconds.

Rotational Spine Stretch

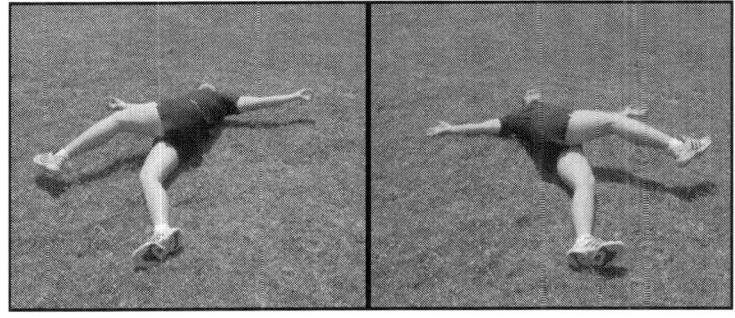

- Start in the supine position with the arms at the "T" position.
- Keeping the arms on the ground, slowly cross one leg over the other and rotate the trunk to move the foot toward the opposite hand.
- Perform slow movements from side to side. Pause only briefly at end range rather than holding as a static stretch.
- The hand can be used to gently pull the crossed leg slightly farther.
- Perform 3-5 repetitions.

Prayer Stretch with Diagonals

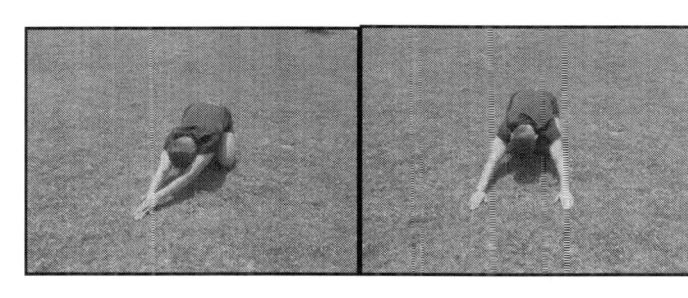

- Move from the Prone Press directly to the prayer stretch, leaving the arms as far forward as possible and sitting back on the heels.
- The head should be down and the back muscles relaxed. This exercise can be used as a motion exercise by taking just a brief pause at end range, or it can be held for 15-30 seconds like a traditional stretch.
- Return to the Prone Press, then repeat with diagonal prayer stretches by crossing the left hand over right, then right over left.
- Hold for 10 seconds.

Hip Flexor Stretch

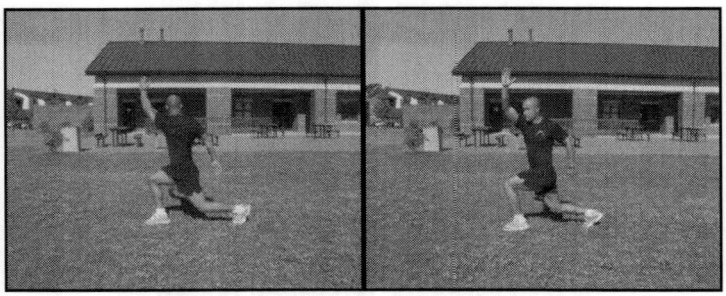

- This stretch uses the same technique as the Walking Lunge and Reach from Movement Prep
- Perform a full forward lunge, keeping the trunk upright and the abs tight. It may also improve the stretch by contracting the glutes on the side of the stretch.
- Rotate the trunk toward the side of the forward leg and sink into the lunge position. A stretch should be felt in the hip flexors of the rear leg.
- Hold for at least 15 seconds.

Hamstring Stretch

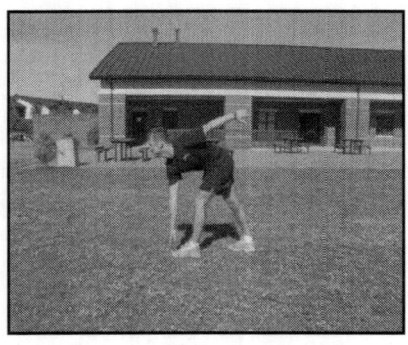

- This stretch uses the same technique as the Walking Bend and Reach from Movement Prep.
- Step forward with the leg while bending forward at the waist.
- Keep the trunk as straight as possible while reaching toward the opposite foot.
- The front knee should flex only slightly. A gentle stretch should be felt in the hamstring of the forward leg. Stop as soon as the stretch is felt.
- Hold for at least 15 seconds.

2-Part Calf Stretch

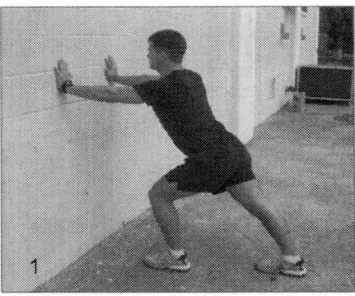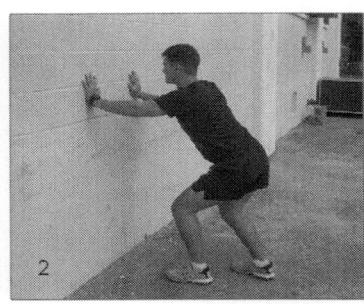

- Use either a wall or a partner to create greater leverage for this stretch.
- For part one, the feet are directed straight toward the wall/partner. The back knee is straight, the heel is down and the pelvis is pushed forward. The stretch should be felt in the upper portion of the back of the calf of the rearward leg.
- For part two, the back leg is brought closer to the wall, the knee is bent, and the body is lowered to create a stretch on the lower portion of the calf of the back leg.
- Hold for at least 15 seconds.

Pec Stretch

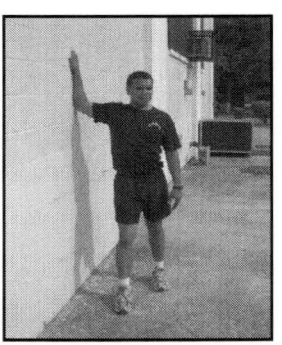

- Use either a wall or a partner to create greater leverage for this stretch.
- Place the forearm on the wall (lock hands and forearms if using the partner method), and turn slowly away until a stretch is felt in the chest. The leg on the stretch side is forward.
- Ensure that the stretch is felt in the Pec muscle, not the shoulder joint. Leaning into the wall/partner and changing the arm elevation (up or down) will transfer the stretch from the joint to the muscles.
- Hold for at least 15 seconds

Strength Training

- Schedule 3 different strength workouts for every 7-10 day period: one heavy resistance workout, one power/power-endurance workout, and one muscular endurance workout.

- Leaders must ensure that every Ranger masters form for every strength training exercise.

- All functional strength training is core training…engage your core before and throughout every lift.

- The heavy resistance workout is based on the 4-rep max. This means that the fourth rep is completed with perfect form.

- The heavy resistance workout must balance pushing, pulling, and multi-joint exercises. Don't over-emphasize the bench press.

- For the power/power-endurance workouts (Ground Base, cleans, Tabata intervals, etc.), don't add so much weight or so many reps that the speed of movement is compromised. Basically this means that the speed with which the movement is initiated is maintained until completion of the movement…or "start fast, finish fast."

- There are dozens of variations on the muscular endurance workout. If you are alternating pushing, pulling, legs, and core, you are meeting the intent.

Methodology for RAW Strength Training

No one questions the notion that Rangers should be strong. The questions are:
- What type of strength do we need?
- How strong do we need to be?
- How do we get that strong with limited time and equipment?

Strength is the ability to overcome resistance. The types of strength that Rangers need fall in to three basic categories:

1. Body Weight:
   o This starts with the ability to stabilize the main joints involved in an exercise so that movement is smooth and efficient rather than sloppy. Once you can stabilize, then build muscular endurance by increasing the volume of training (sets x reps) for exercises like push-ups, pull-ups, single-leg squats, lunges, and a variety of core exercises.

2. Heavy External Resistance:
   o This type of strength is needed to move loads. You must first be able to stabilize the joints used in the movement, but you don't have to wait until you've built up a given level of body-weight muscular endurance. Moderate to heavy lifting can begin early in a program as long as form is good and stability is maintained.

3. Power/Power Endurance:
   o This type of strength moves a load rapidly. The load may be your own body (ex: jumping onto an elevated platform) or an external load (ex: hoisting equipment onto an elevated platform). Power training is more demanding on the neuromuscular and skeletal systems, so stability, correct form, and adequate recovery are essential.

How strong do Rangers need to be? As with the other components of physical fitness, strength is useful to the extent that it improves your performance and keeps you injury free. There is no requirement to look like a bodybuilder or hoist weight like an Olympian. For Rangers, strength means being able to carry your combat load indefinitely, being able to carry the wounded man next to you, being able to get in the window or up the rope…These tasks and the many others Rangers will encounter require broad-spectrum strength.

For performance oriented strength training, the goal is the movement rather than the muscle. For example, a bodybuilder wanting to develop the quadriceps muscles may isolate that group on a machine that resists the straightening of the legs. The goal is muscular development and a visually pleasing shape. The bodybuilder is not concerned about the movement that caused the development. Contrast this with Rangers who, like athletes, need leg strength for lifting, lunging, climbing, and jumping. Now the concern is for the power of the movement, not the size or appearance of the muscle.

It is common to hear a strength coach describe an athlete that can step into a squat rack and work with more than 500 pounds, but can't do one correct single-leg squat with just their body weight. The difference is the much greater balance and stability demands of the single-leg squat. Balance and stability, especially of the core, are essential for developing functional strength. Informed athletes know that without a strong core their performance will suffer and they are more susceptible to injury. Top strength and conditioning coaches spend much more time emphasizing work on this area than on glamour exercises like the bench press and biceps curl.

The importance of the core is due to its relationship with the limbs. The core must be stable so that the limbs have a fixed base from which to create powerful movements. Without a strong, stable base of support, trying to generate power from the arms and legs is like pushing an object while on ice (or firing cannon from a canoe). The core is stabilized by a ring of muscles that loop around the spine and connect it to the pelvis. Even muscles like the glutes and lats play a big role via their attachments to the spine and pelvis. You are only as strong as your weakest link. Maxing the sit-up event doesn't mean you can stabilize the trunk. In fact there is evidence that concentrating on the sit-up and ignoring the other muscle groups can actually hinder your ability to stabilize the core. We must train 360-degree abdominal/trunk strength, and in a manner that mimics the core's function.

Rangers just starting a resistance training program can get significantly stronger in just a few sessions, even before muscle mass increases. This is due to the fact that they have become more proficient at recruiting muscle fibers for the task. If we never attempt to meet heavy resistance, these nerve-to-muscle messages may not be very efficient. This is a common flaw in PT programs geared toward the APFT.

With heavy resistance, form becomes very important for both performance and safety. You must teach your soldiers safe lifting techniques and see them demonstrate correct lifts with a light weight. Realize that heavy resistance training for a given movement will require more rest (generally, about 48 hours) between bouts of exercise than will muscular endurance training.

Form is also important at lower levels of resistance. When we train for muscular endurance, changes are taking place at the cellular level that allow the working muscles to sustain their work for longer periods of time. Repetitions, by definition, are high for muscular endurance training. With repetition comes muscle memory, so form becomes very important toward ensuring that we "memorize" the correct movement.

It should come as no surprise that correct form is also a requirement for effective power training. In fact, creating optimal power is impossible without biomechanically-correct technique. Rangers should train across the power and power-endurance spectrum. For power, keep the rep range below five, adjusting the weight accordingly. Remember, power is about force production and rate of movement…so move the weight fast. Contrast this with heavy dead lifting, which involves relatively slow movement. For power-endurance, the weight decreases to 50-60% of 1RM or below.

In the RAW program, Ground Base equipment has been the primary tool for developing power-endurance. When used for power-endurance, keep the loads light enough that the speed of movement is not sacrificed. Resist the temptation to focus on the amount of weigh and instead focus on form and power. Ground

Base is by no means the only way to train power-endurance. Any form of resistance that allows controlled, rapid movement can be used.

Execution of RAW Strength Training

Muscular Endurance Workout

Purpose: Develop control of body weight from the ground, on the feet and from the air (pull up bar, ropes). Improve total body muscular endurance.

Utilization: This workout should be performed at least once during every 7-10 day period. Sessions should be completed in about 30 minutes. It is easily combined with a tempo run or 300-yard shuttle repeats for a complete PT session. This workout can be performed indoors or outdoors.

Execution: Perform the exercises in the order listed below. Perform all sets of each exercise before moving to the next. Emphasize mastery of exercise technique first, and then gradually introduce more challenging movements (see progression below). Resistance can also be added once body-weight exercise becomes easy. This can be as easy as performing the workout in kit, holding dumbbells/barbell plates/sandbags, etc.

Exercises

- Single-leg Squat (2 sets, 15 reps each leg; adjust depth as needed)
- Pull-Ups/Ropes Tng (2 sets of 12 reps; partner or elastic band assistance as needed)
- Core (Supine Bicycle and/or Supine Twist (1 set, 1 minute)
- Single-leg Stiff-leg Deadlift (1 set, 15 reps each leg; adjust range-of-motion as needed)
- Nordic Hamstring (Kneeling w/partner hold at ankle; use pads at knees as needed; 1 set of 15 reps)
- Push-ups (1 Ranger pushing, 1 spotting; perform 3 sets at 60, 40, and 30 seconds each)
- Hanging Crunches/Heel Claps (2 sets of 12 reps; partner assistance as needed)
- Star Lunge Series (2 sets of 5 reps each direction – see execution note below)
- Pull-ups/Push-ups (1 set each, max good reps with only transitional rest in between)
- Core (Planks, Side-planks)

Note 1: If medicine balls are available, parts of the MedBall drill can be used in place of sit-ups, supine bicycle/twist.

Note 2: Perform the Star Lunge Series as follows: 1) Left leg forward, forward-diagonal, lateral; 2) Right leg forward, forward-diagonal, lateral; 3) Left leg lateral, backward-diagonal, rear (reaching with right leg), 4) Right leg lateral, backward-diagonal, rear (reaching with left leg). 5) Repeat all of the above for a second set.

Progression

- Add resistance to single-leg exercises/lunges (med balls, dumbbells/kettlebells, plates, and pull-ups (RBA).
- Combine forward and rear lunges. For example, perform a forward lunge with the left leg then pass the starting position without stopping to go into a rear lunge in which the left leg steps back, but the weight remains on the right leg. Repeat for one minute, rest 30 seconds, and then repeat for the opposite side. Use the first three reps to establish form, and then continue at a moderate to fast pace.
- 3-Point Pushup (60-40-30s sets with 60-40-30s rest; 1 Ranger pushing, 1 spotting)

Alternatives

- There are plenty of alternatives to the muscular endurance workout described above. When evaluating other routines, look for the following:
  - pushing and pulling movements for the upper body
  - a variety of core exercises targeting different areas
  - a variety of functional leg exercises (squats, lunges, single-leg step-ups)

- a reasonable volume of training (a workout that calls for 50 reps when you can only do 20 good reps is not reasonable)

- a reasonable load based on your individual abilities, not what some guy with a website has published as "the standard"

- a reasonable degree of recovery built into the workout (you should feel like your stamina is being challenged throughout the workout, but not so much that movements become sloppy…take short breaks as needed to regain some energy)

Single-Leg Squat

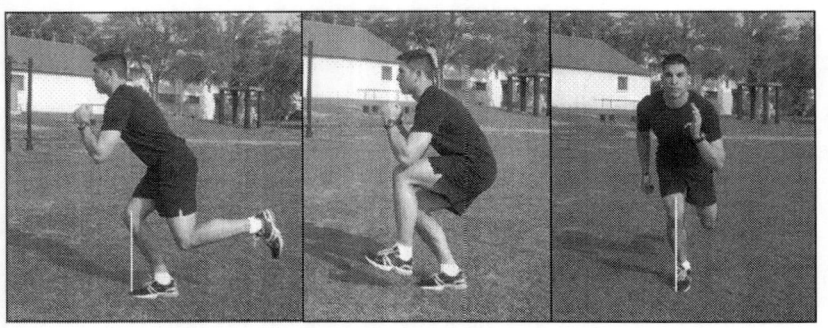

- Perform 2 sets of 15 reps for each leg.
- Squat as low as possible without breaking form, then pause for 1-2 seconds. Return smoothly to the starting position.
- At the bottom of the squat, the knee must be aligned directly over the ball of the foot (note the alignment markers in the pictures above. The back should be straight, but the trunk is tilted forward to counterbalance the rearward movement of the hips.

Single Leg Stiff-Leg Deadlift

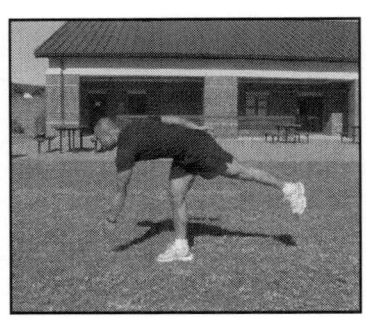

- Stand on one leg. Keeping the trunk straight, lean forward and reach toward the opposite foot as the free leg is raised in line with the trunk.
- The stance knee is slightly bent and remains in that position throughout the exercise.
- Perform 1 set of 15 reps on each leg, using slow, controlled movements.
-

Pull-Ups/Chin-Ups/Ropes

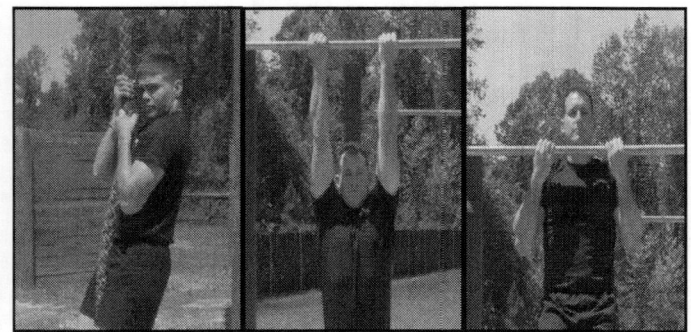

- In buddy teams, perform 2 sets of 12 reps, alternating pull-ups, chin-ups, or rope pulls.
- Do not kip; use partner assistance as needed.
- Return to the straight arm position after each repetition.

Nordic Hamstring

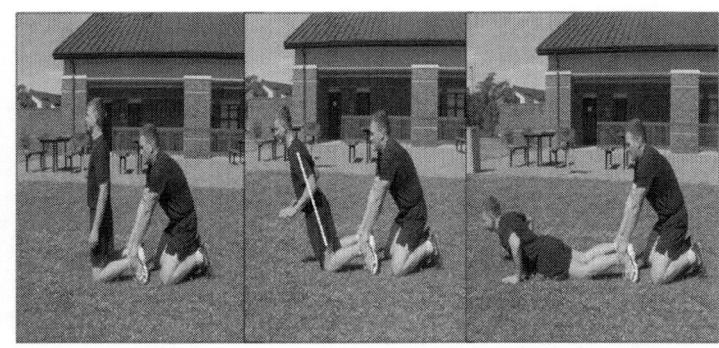

- Perform in buddy teams as shown above; 1 set of 15 progressive reps.
- Do not bend at the waist; keep the trunk and thighs lined up as shown in the second picture.
- The first few repetitions involve leaning forward without going to the ground. Once you reach an angle from which you are unable to return to the starting position, allow the straight trunk to fall forward and use a plyo push-up to return to the starting position.

Push-Ups

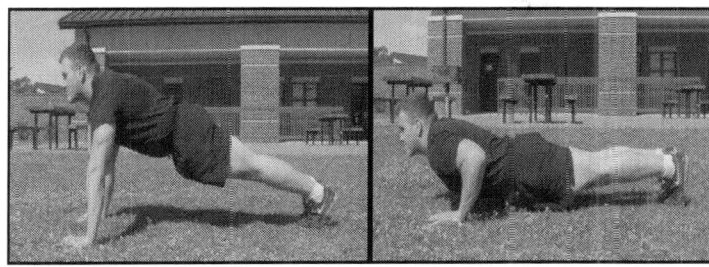

- 1 Ranger pushing, 1 spotting; perform 3 sets at 60, 40, and 30 seconds each
- Do not rest or move out of a tight front-leaning-rest position; spotters assist as needed with the minimal amount of lift at the waist.

Star Lunges

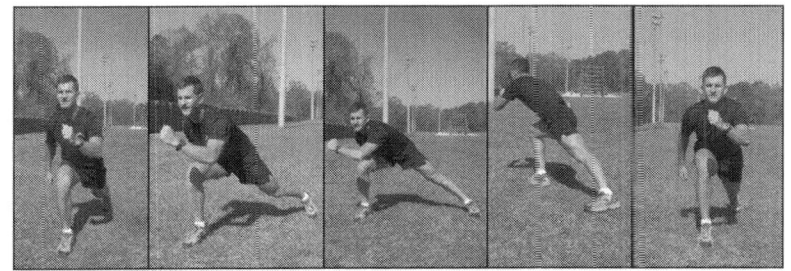

Forward   Front Diagonal   Lateral   Back Diagonal   Rear

- Perform 5 reps each in order: 1) Left leg forward, front-diagonal, lateral; 2) Right leg forward, front-diagonal, lateral; 3) Left leg lateral, backward-diagonal, rear (reaching with right leg), 4) Right leg lateral, backward-diagonal, rear (reaching with left leg). 5) Repeat all of the above for a second set.
- For every repetition, the knee of the working leg (left leg in first 4 pictures above, right leg in last picture) should be aligned directly above the ball of the foot at the end range position. Push vigorously from the working leg to return to the starting position; do not jerk the trunk.
- Pivot on the ball of the plant foot (right foot in pictures above) and point the toes in the direction of the lunge to avoid twisting through the knee.

Hanging Crunches / Heels

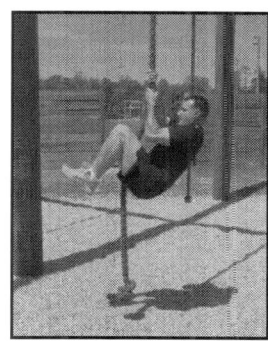

- Can be performed from a bar or rope
- Perform 2 sets of 12 reps in buddy teams; one spotter, one executing.
- Maintain the flexed-elbow position and lift the knees to the elbows. Spotters assist as needed on the "up" phase of the exercise.
- Maintain control throughout the exercise- do not let the body sway back and forth, or use momentum to get knees up.
- An advanced technique on the pull-up bar is to tap the heels over the bar.

Supine Bicycle

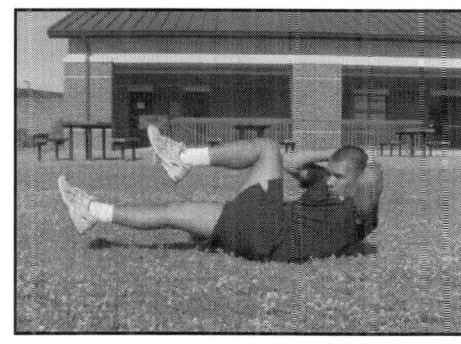

- Perform 1 set for 1 minute.
- Perform at a slow pace without jerking on the neck.
- Attempt to touch the elbow to the opposite knee.
- Reach as far as possible with the straight leg and lower it slowly to within a few inches of the ground.
- Do not allow the low back to arch off the ground.

Heavy Resistance Workout

Purpose: Develop total-body muscular strength. This is not meant to be a body-builder's workout. Lifts that involve multiple joints and muscle groups are the standard.

Utilization: Generally once every 7-10 days in all phases.

Execution: There are two main options for strength training - the gym-based method and the field-expedient method.

- Gym-Based Method: Execution depends on the time available.

1. No time constraint

   The following guidelines apply if you have plenty of time for strength training (deployed, split PT sessions, etc).

   - Over the course of a week, balance upper and lower body lifting
   - Over the course of a week, balance push and pull lifting
   - Work the upper body 1-3x/week
   - Work the legs 1-2x/week
   - Each month, change the workout in some way. One option is to change the lifts (Ex. Switch from seated row to single-arm bent-over rows.) Another option is to switch from heavy resistance (based on a 4-rep max) with relatively long recovery between sets to an 8-10-rep max with a relatively short recovery. Another options is to superset (one example is to immediately follow a push lift with a pull exercise)
   - If performing split routines, they should be arranged according to push/pull functions. For example one day chest and triceps, the next day back and biceps. Because the stabilizers of the shoulder are highly stressed during a chest workout, avoid a hard isolated shoulder workout the day before or after the chest. It's probably best to work the shoulders on chest day as part of the pushing function. Keep in mind that this type of training that isolates muscle groups is not necessary for functional strength. Though some Rangers may benefit from increasing their overall mass with such routines, they must supplement these routines with functional, total-body movements.
   - Your max bench press should not be considered the most important measure of your strength. Most of the time when you have to push something heavy, you will get your legs into it. That's why we prefer Ground Base, push press with dumbbells, dead lifts, squats, and other total body lifts. Heavy benching also carries a risk of injury to the shoulder, both for pec and rotator cuff strains/tears and long-term degeneration. If you have any doubt about your risk with heavy pressing movement, see your local physical therapist.

2. Time Constraint
   If all squads from a given company are performing this session during the same time period (a typical garrison, 90-minute AM PT session), then strength training needs to be limited to about 20 minutes per platoon in order to accommodate three platoons in one hour. For example, after movement prep, the squads from first platoon have the weight room for 20 minutes, while squads from the other platoons are on the field doing something else. The squads rotate at 20 and 40 minutes. The 20-minute sessions proceed as follows:

- Perform a warm-up set at about 50% of 4-rep max.
- Perform the second set at about 75% of 4-rep max.
- Perform 2 sets at 4-rep max. Adjust the weight so that the fourth rep is the last rep that can be completed with perfect form. Do not continue to muscle failure or allow a repetition that involves jerking or other compensatory movements. Each set will last about 15-20 seconds. Each individual should have 60 seconds rests between sets, for a 1:3-4 work-to-rest ratio. Finish all sets before moving to the next station.

Notes:

- In the Legs/Back and Pull categories, change lifts after 4-5 sessions. For example, Rangers that have been performing the Deadlift and Seated Cable Row might switch to the Stiff-leg Deadlift and Lat Pull-down.
- Pre-position weights to allow time-efficient changing out of weights for lifts that use barbells/dumbbells. Remember, there will generally only be about 6-7 minutes per station.

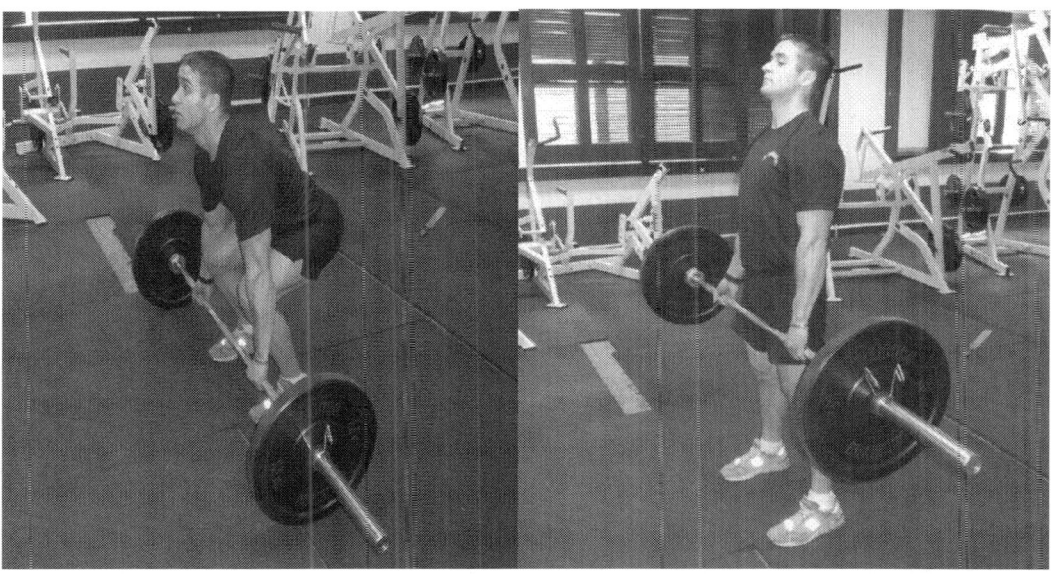

For the barbell deadlift, the feet are under the bar, the back straight, shoulders pulled back and aligned over the bar, heels down, hips low, head and chest up, and arms outside the legs. Breathe in and hold, push through the heels to rise to a fully upright stance. Breathe out as you pass through the most difficult part of the lift. Keep the bar as close to the body as possible. Attempt to rise as a unit rather than using the hips first and then the upper body. There is no need to lean backward at the top.

- Field-Expedient Method:

1. The principles of strength training used in the weight room still apply when conducting field-expedient strength training. In other words, push and pull, work upper and lower body. Resistance comes from your body weight, your kit, sandbags, kettle bells, etc.

2. Working push strength means adding a challenge to the standard pushup. There are many ways to do this: 3-point PU, wearing your rack, partner resistance, elastic band resistance, elevated PU (partner holds your feet at his waist level), partner puts a sandbag on your back, or any combination of the above.

3. Working pull strength is straight forward. Perform pull-ups, chin-ups, alternating grip pull-ups…perform in kit for progression. Also perform ropes training without the use of your legs. Use dip bars to perform horizontal pulls (partner holds your feet or you hook them over the dip bars).

4.   Leg strength can be trained with tire flips, partner carries, log drills, weighted lunges/split-squats, single-leg squats, and step-ups. Add weight through kit, sandbags, etc. To perform step ups, first identify an appropriate height. When the foot is placed on the step, your thigh should be roughly parallel with the ground. Perform by placing one leg on the step, leaning forward, powering up with the lead leg only, and then slowly lowering the body to just barely touch the back leg down.

Perform several sets of exercises in each category. Add resistance when perfect form can be held for 12 or more reps.

Power and Power-Endurance Workouts
Ground Base Equipment

Purpose: Develop total body power-endurance using functional movements.

Utilization: Once or twice per week in all phases. If the BN is scheduling one company per day to use the Ground Base equipment, then this session should last no more than 20 minutes in order to accommodate three platoons in one hour. Even when used in small groups without time constraint, an effective circuit(s) can be completed in 15-30 minutes.

Execution:

1) This first option assumes battalion-level scheduling to maximize use of the Ground Base equipment. Battalions should provide 3 stations for each of the six lifts listed below. Arrange the weight room for ease of transition. For battalions that use the rotating schedule and dedicate a company per day for the Ground Base workout, it is best to set up the machines in advance – one set of machines each at light, medium, and heavy levels of resistance. Platoons are sent through one at a time, switching out at 20 minutes. There are 2 Rangers at each station – 1 performing and 1 resting. After both Rangers have completed the lift, move to the next station. Complete the entire circuit twice, with a 2-3 minute break between iterations. During this break, switch the weights for the Combo Incline and Combo Decline in order to work the opposite side. Do not perform any of the Ground Base lifts to muscle failure or allow a repetition that involves jerking or other compensatory movements. The primary means of progression is through speed of movement and increased duration of sets. Initially (Phase 1) adjust the weight so that 20 seconds of work can be completed with perfect form. Progress by either adding weight or performing for 30 seconds (Phases 2 & 3). For larger elements, 3 Rangers per station may be necessary to finish in 20 minutes. Under those circumstances, continue to use 20-second work cycles.

<u>The Six Stations:</u>

R Combo Twist
L Combo Twist
Combo Incline (1st Set L, 2nd Set R)
Combo Decline (1st Set L, 2nd Set R)
Zero Woodchopper Up (1st Set L, 2nd Set R)
Jammer

2) When performing a Ground Base workout individually or in small groups with no time/equipment constraints, you need not use the circuit method described above. One option is to use the Tabata interval method, using 20s of work followed by 10s of rest, with 8 repetitions (total of four minutes). There are numerous variations using Ground Base. We suggest dedicating a Tabata round (4 minutes) alternating left and right movements for two lifts (combo twist, woodchopper up, incline/decline, etc). The round should be followed by several minutes rest, then a second round using another lift. Repeat until all desired lifts are completed or until fatigue sacrifices movement speed/proficiency.

You can also adjust the sets/reps to stress power more than power-endurance. For example, once you have mastered form, add enough weight to decrease the reps to the 3-5 rep range. Do not add so much weight that speed of movement is lost…remember this is a power workout. To maintain precision of movement with this heavier load, allow adequate recovery between sets (generally 1-3 minutes).

Right Combo Twist

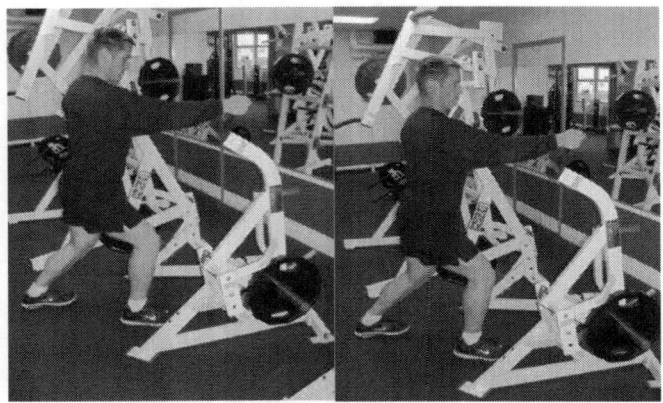

- Start in the power stance crouch with the left leg forward. The core muscles should be contracted and ready.
- Power the movement by rising out of the crouch, twisting through pelvis and trunk, and finishing with the arm movements.
- Reverse and complete the **Left Combo Twist**

Combo Decline

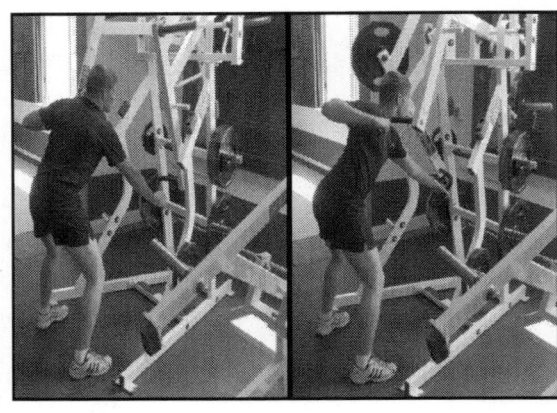

- For the left combo decline, start in the power stance crouch with the left leg forward. The parallel stance position is an alternative and is shown in the 2 pictures on the right. The core muscles should be contracted and ready.
- Power the movement by twisting through pelvis and trunk, and pushing/pulling with the arms.
- Perform an equal number of left and right combo incline sets.

Combo Incline

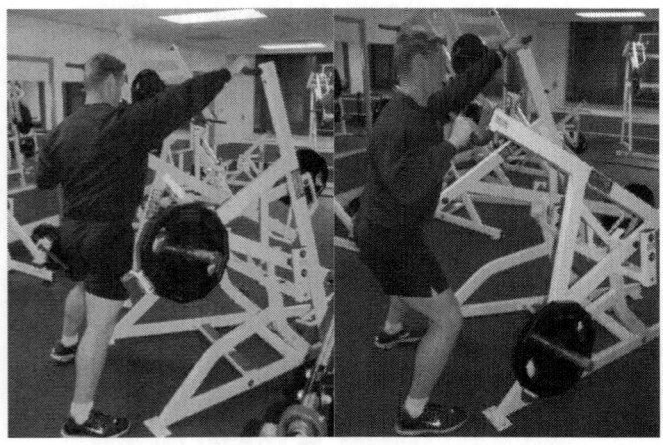

- For the left combo incline, start in the power stance crouch with the left leg forward. The core muscles should be contracted and ready.
- Power the movement by rising forcefully out of the crouch, twisting through pelvis and trunk, and finishing with the arm movements.
- Perform an equal number of left and right combo incline sets.

Jammer

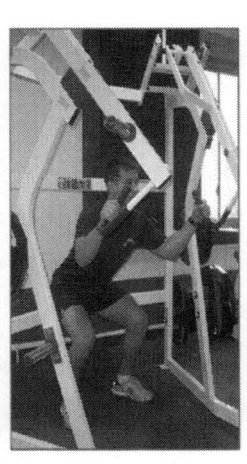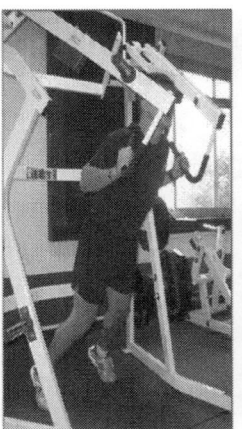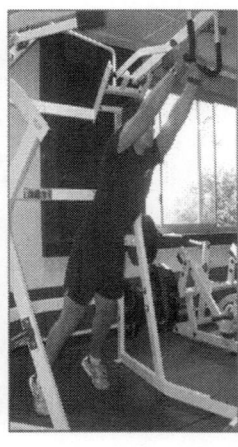

- Start in a power stance crouch, with the feet parallel. The core muscles should be contracted and ready.
- Power the lift with an explosive push through the legs, finishing with the pressing movement. The trunk must remain straight at all times.
- If motion stops midway or the spine arches, either the weight is too heavy or the technique has not been mastered.

Zero Wood Chopper Up

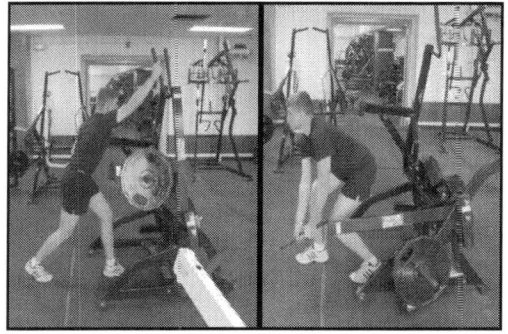

- Start in a well-balanced crouch, either facing the handle or angled slightly away from the machine. The back is straight, and the head and chest are up. The core muscles should be contracted and ready.
- Power the lift with an explosive push through the legs, creating enough momentum so that you can pivot on the balls of the feet during the mid-range.
- Finish by releasing the lower hand and guiding the weight up with a pressing motion keeping the back straight and the abdominals engaged.

Squat High Pull

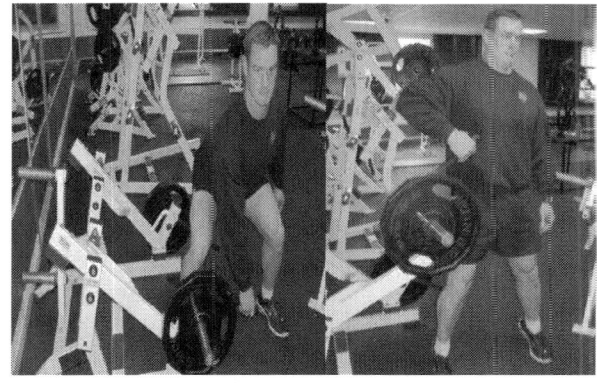

- Begin in a deep squat with heels down, back straight, core muscles tight and head and chest up. Grasp bar with
- Take a deep breath in and hold it. Explode out of the squat by pushing through the heels. Keep the back straight and chest high.
- Momentum should take weight to chest level. Hand should act as a brake to keep weight from going past chest.

Ground Base Deadlift

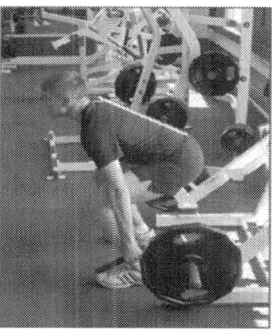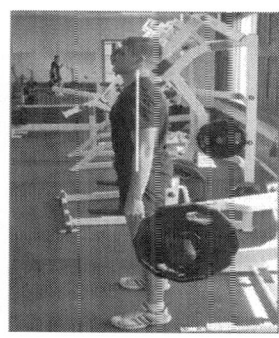

- Begin in a deep squat with heels down, back straight, core muscles tight and head and chest up.
- Take a deep breath in and hold it. Rise out of the squat by pushing through the heels. Keep the back straight and chest high.
- Release the breath once after clearing the most difficult part of the lift (sticking point).
- Do not arch the back at the end of the lift. This is only necessary for competition.

Ground Base Stiff-Leg Deadlift

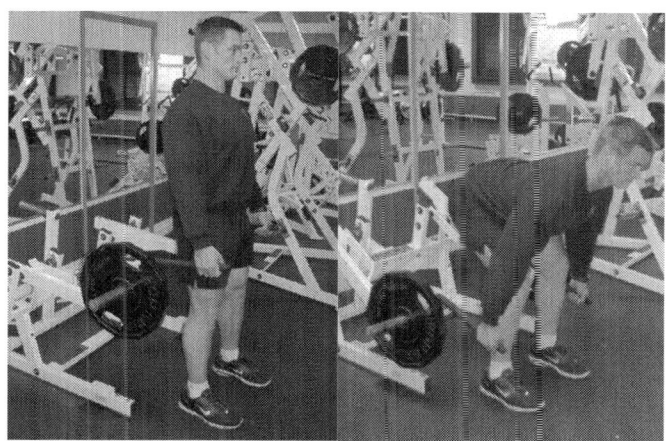

- The Ground Base Deadlift station is recommended for all inexperienced lifters
- Begin with the heels down, back straight, core muscles tight, and head and chest up. Knees are only slightly flexed.
- Take a deep breath in and hold it. Rise out of the squat by pushing through the heels. Keep the back straight and chest high.
- Release the breath once after clearing the most difficult part of the lift (sticking point).
- Do not arch the back at the end of the lift.

Power Drill

Purpose: Develop total body power/power-endurance using functional movements.

Utilization: Perform 2-3x/month, beginning after mastery of jump/land biomechanics. This drill is best performed immediately after movement prep.

Execution:

The first time this drill is performed, the movements must be taught, so there may not be much of a training effect other than learning. Emphasis is on correct execution, not creating a smoke session. The work-to-rest ratio should begin at about 1:4 for each exercise. Add speed/intensity and shorter recovery only after the basic skill is mastered.

The foundational movement for all jumps is the power position, with hips to the rear, knees over feet, heels down, back straight but trunk tilting forward. Body weight is primarily on the balls of the feet. Landings should be soft, with impact absorbed by plenty of bend of the hips and knees. Keep the feet shoulder width apart or less. Do not allow the knees to buckle inward or outward upon landing.

For the med ball throws, perform in pairs, with two ranks facing. For safety purposes, it is best to only throw on command from the squad leader, with throws going from one rank to another rather than randomly. See the individual drills below for details.

Exercises:

o Sprints: Build to an 80-90% effort over the first 20 yards, then maintain for a total of 60-80 yards. Rest for 15-30 seconds. Perform 6-10 reps.
o Broad Jump: 3 w/pause, then 7 continuous; repeat 2-3X
o Lateral Hop, Double-leg over cone: max # in 10s, 40s rest, then repeat
o Modified Squat Jumper: 3 w/pause between reps, then 8-10 continuous
o Split-Squat Jump: 8 reps each leg
o Plyo Push-up (8-10 reps with partner assist as needed)
o 90/180 Jumps: 3 w/pause, then 8-10 continuous
o MedBall Throws for Distance (underhand, backward-overhead, chest push, rotation L/R)

Optional Progression

o Scissors Jump w/rotation (in place of Split-Squat Jump): Sprint 10M after 5th rep. Add MedBall only if perfect execution

Power Drill Sprints

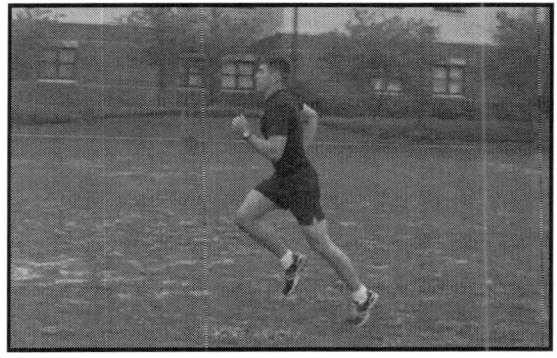

- Build to an 80-90% effort over the first 20 yards, then maintain for a total of 60-80 yards. Rest for 15-30 seconds. Perform 6-10 reps.

Power Drill—Lateral Hop

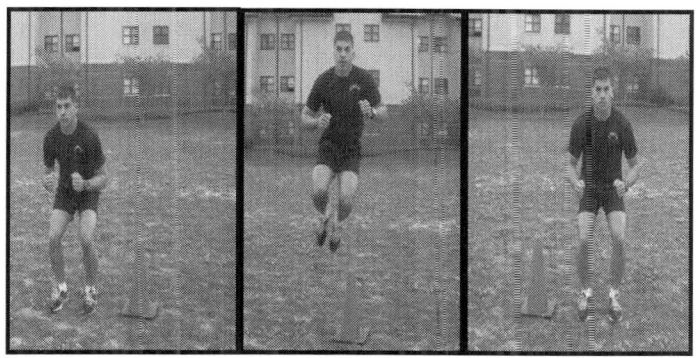

- Perform double-leg jumps over cones. Note that the feet remain within about 6 inches apart and directed forward.
- Perform the maximum number of reps in 10 seconds. Rest 40 seconds, then repeat.

Power Drill—Broad Jump

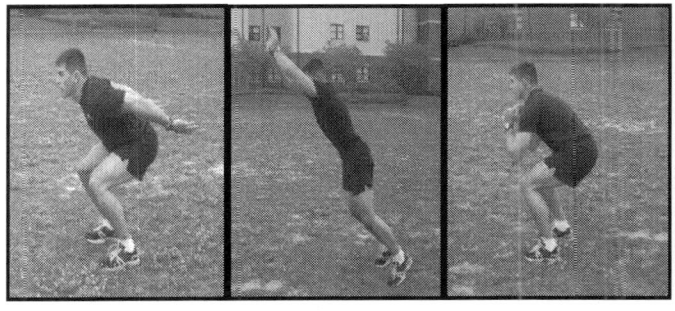

- Start and finish in the power position.
- Stick the landing and pause for the first 3 jumps, then perform 5 continuous jumps
- Repeat 2-3X

Power Drill-Modified BURPEE

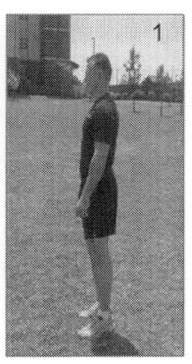
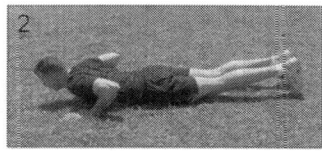
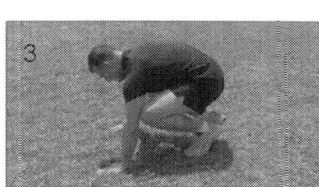
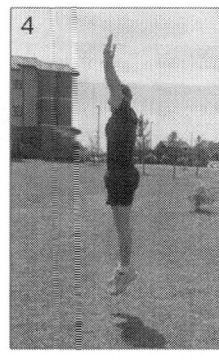

- From a regular stance (1) perform a modified squat thrust. Do not stop in the front leaning rest position. Instead drop directly into position 2 above.
- Jump quickly into the power position (3) and, without pause, jump forcefully, extending the arms overhead (4).
- Land back in the power position (3). Stick the landing and return to the starting position for the first 3 reps, then perform 8-10 continuous reps. For the continuous reps, do not return to the starting position between reps.

Power Drill—Split Squat Jump

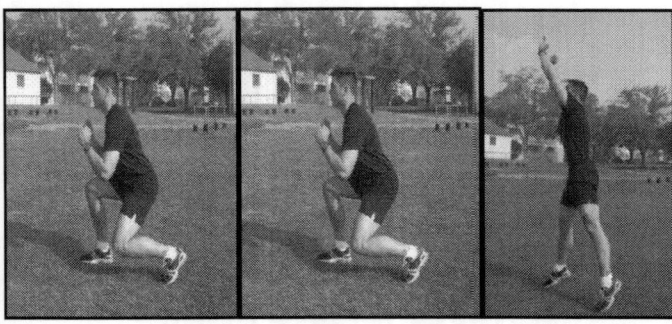

- From a staggered stance, with 80% of body-weight on the front leg, jump vigorously and extend the arms overhead.
- Land softly back in the starting position by getting plenty of impact absorption from the bending of the hips and knees.

Power Drill—90-180 Jumps

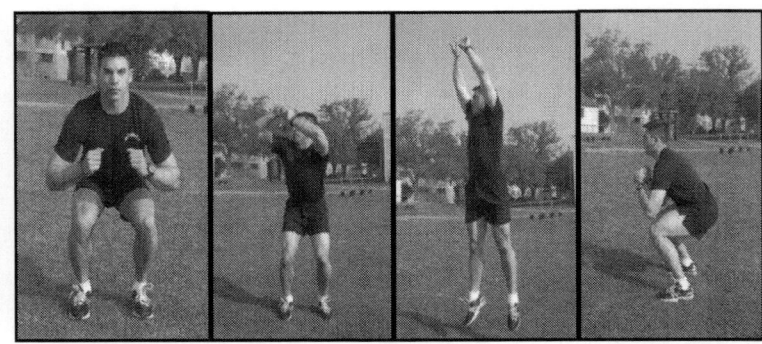

- From the power stance, jump vigorously and extend the arms overhead while rotating the body 90 degrees to the right.
- Land softly by getting plenty of impact absorption from the bending of the hips and knees. Continue with several jumps clockwise, attempting to land at exactly the 90-degree mark. Repeat in the counter-clockwise direction. Progress to 180 degree jumps.

Power Drill—Plyometric Push-up

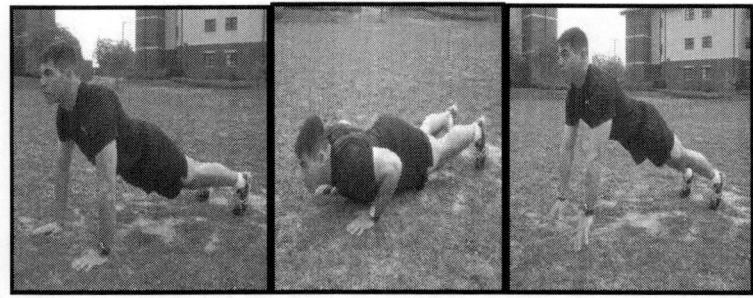

- Start in the front leaning rest position. Drop quickly to within a few inches of the ground, then explode upward with enough force that the hands leave the ground
- Do not pause in the front leaning rest once you begin the exercise.
- Maintain a tight core throughout.
- Perform 2 sets of 8-10 reps with partner assist as needed.

Power Drill
Scissor Jump with Rotation

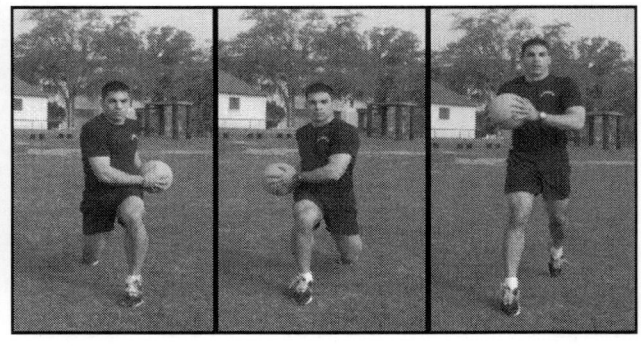

- From a staggered stance, with 80% of body-weight on the front leg and the med ball held to the outside of the front thigh, jump vigorously and swing the ball to the opposite side while "scissoring" the legs.
- Land softly by getting plenty of impact absorption from the bending of the hips and knees.

MED BALL THROW
Underhand

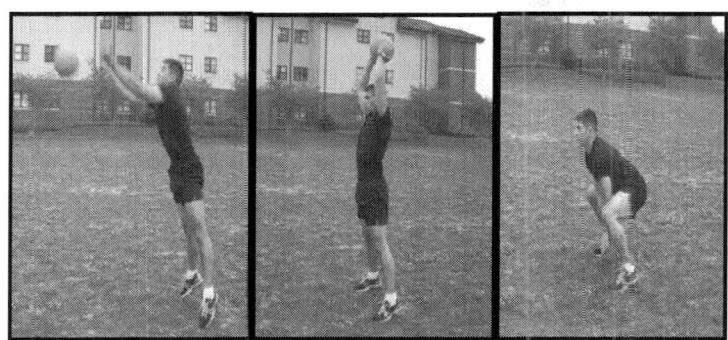

- Raise the ball overhead, then quickly drop into the power position with the arms extended.
- Without pause, explode out of the power position to throw the ball in a 45-degree arc. You should land 2-3 feet in front of the starting position.
- This drill is normally performed with a partner about 20 yards away, positioned to catch the ball on one bounce. Do not attempt to catch in the air.

MED BALL THROW
Chest Push

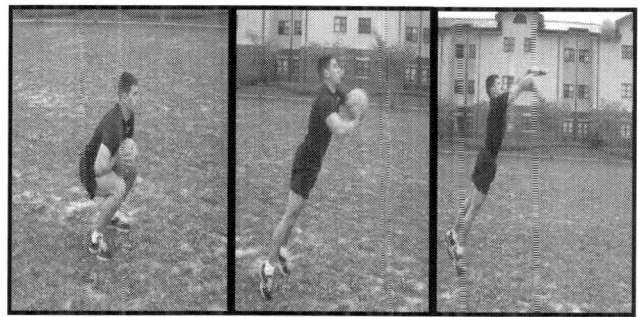

- Pull the ball into the chest as you squat.
- Without pause, explode out of the power position to throw the ball in a 45-degree arc. You should land 2-3 feet in front of the starting position.
- This drill is normally performed with a partner about 15 yards away, positioned to catch the ball on one bounce. Do not attempt to catch in the air. When performed in larger groups, it is best to have one rank at a time throw on command.

MED BALL THROW
Backward Over-Head

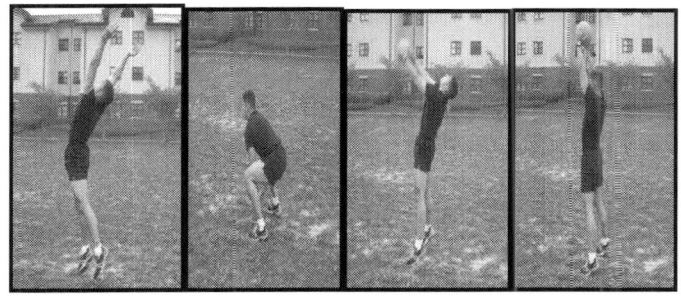

- Raise the ball overhead, then quickly drop into the power position with the arms extended.
- Without pause, explode out of the power position to throw the ball in a 45-degree arc overhead.
- This drill is normally performed with a partner about 20 yards away, positioned to catch the ball on one bounce. Do not attempt to catch in the air.

MED BALL THROW
Rotation Left/Right

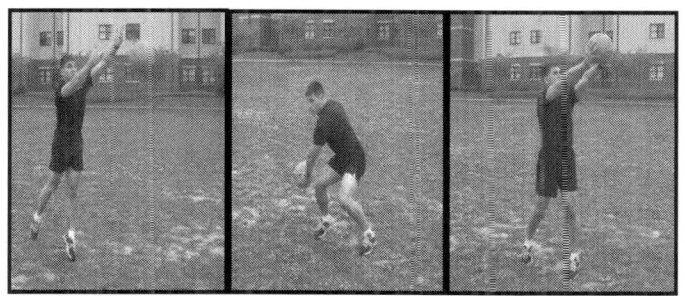

- Raise the ball overhead toward your partner, then quickly drop into the rotated power position with the arms extended (middle photo)
- Without pause, explode out of the this position to throw the ball in a 45-degree arc. You should land 1-2 feet in front of the starting position. Perform an equal number of R/L throws.
- This drill is normally performed with a partner about 20 yards away, positioned to catch the ball on one bounce. Do not attempt to catch in the air. When performed in larger groups, it is best to have one rank at a time throw on command.

Other Power and Power-Endurance Workouts

- **Tabata Intervals** are named after the author of a famous study that proved high-intensity intervals of short duration (20s), with an even shorter rest (10s), repeated 8 times, could significantly improve *both* anaerobic and aerobic endurance over six weeks (5x/week). These results were compared to a group that trained at a steady pace for one hour, 5X/week at 70% of aerobic capacity. The steady-pace, moderate intensity training did not improve anaerobic capacity. While the Tabata research was performed on a cycle ergometer, a similar effect can be had performing a variety of powerful movements using body weight and/or external resistance. There are several possible applications of Tabata intervals within RAW. A single round (20s work, 10s rest x 8 reps = 4 minutes) can easily be combined with another "main" training event. Even two rounds with a 2-minute rest between rounds only demands 10 minutes. There are dozens of potential exercises that can be used for Tabata intervals. We like the following:

  - Modified Burpees
  - MedBall (Short and Medium Range Throws)
  - Suicides (25m x3 equals roughly 20 seconds…adjust according to your speed)
  - Squat Thrusters
  - Tire Flips (with or without in/out jumps)
  - Skedco/Sled Pulls
  - Kettle Bell Swings
  - Kettle Bell Pull (20 yards of rope, 50-60 lbs of kettle bell, hand-over-hand pull)
  - Kettle Bell Snatch (Alternating sides each 20s round)

- The **Olympic lifts** (Snatch and Clean and Jerk) are highly specialized lifts that are proven means of increasing power. However, they are technically demanding lifts that when performed incorrectly can lead to injury.

Since there are many other ways to develop power, our guidance is to use these technically demanding training methods with extreme caution. The National Strength and Conditioning Association has a video resource that includes many power-developing lifts. Go to < http://www.nsca-lift.org/videos/displayvideos.asp> for the videos. Do not overestimate your ability. Take the time to master the technique, and then apply the principles of exercise discussed previously. Make sure your gym has lighter plates (10 or 15#) with which to master these techniques (same diameter as the typical 45# plate). Before attempting these drills, Rangers should first spend 2-3 months mastering and then progressing the 360-Core, MedBall, Muscular Endurance, Moderate-Heavy resistance, and Ground Base workouts.

Generally power workout incorporate several sets of 3-5 repetitions for each exercise. Sufficient rest between sets ensures that technique remains uncompromised by fatigue. Up to three minutes rest between sets may be necessary. Once the technique is mastered, focus on moving the bar as quickly as possible. Loads of 75-95% of 1RM will result in increased maximum strength, while loads of 50-60% of 1RM, performed ballistically, will result in increased maximum power. Once an athlete has reached high strength levels, maximum power training may be more conducive to peak athletic performance than further increases in max strength.

Principles of Endurance Training

BOTTOM LINE UP FRONT – RAW BULLETS FOR ENDURANCE:

- Schedule 3 different endurance-emphasis workouts for every 7-10 day period.

- Once per week (except on recovery weeks) perform interval training of some sort (30-30s, track intervals, pool intervals, etc).

- Progress time/distance/interval reps by no more than 10% per week.

- Don't run hard and/or long on consecutive days unless you have a good reason for doing so (you are an experienced runner training for a running event).

- During recovery weeks (generally one for every 4 or 5 weeks of hard training), replace intervals, long runs, and foot marches with pool workouts and cardio machines.

Methodology for RAW Endurance Training

For our purposes, endurance is the ability to sustain physical activity. Sometimes the activity is intense and can only be sustained for a relatively short time. With some recovery, the activity can then be repeated. This is anaerobic endurance and is reflective of many combat tasks that involve repeating quick, powerful movements. At other times, the task may be less intense but require continuous movement (ex. a foot movement towards an objective several km away). This type of endurance is aerobic in nature.

Most activities are not purely aerobic or anaerobic, but a mix of the two. Interestingly, training anaerobically will improve aerobic capacity. However, the reverse is not true. For this reason, it is a mistake to train only the aerobic system when missions require full-spectrum endurance.

In the RAW program, endurance is trained primarily through running, footmarches, and swimming. However, it is important to note that an anaerobic training effect is also occurring during many other drills if intensity is maintained. This is especially true with MedBall, agility, and power drills; ground base training; circuits; and Tabata Intervals (described in the Strength section).

To enhance endurance during drills other than running, foot marching, and swimming, reduces the amount of rest time between sets or events. This should only be done after the men have mastered the basic drills. Using the MedBall drill as an example, it is best to keep the relatively long rest time between sets during the initial train up in phase one. This reduces sloppy movement due to fatigue and promotes mastery of the techniques. By phase two, technique should be sufficient to allow a reduction in rest time between sets.

Execution of RAW Endurance Training

1. Sustained-pace run of 30-60 minutes

The purpose of this run is to build aerobic endurance and gradually toughen the legs. In Phase 1, keep the time around 30 minutes. Starting in Phase 2, gradually progress the time/distance based on your needs. A good rule of thumb is to increase running distance by no more than 10 percent per week. Thus, adding about 3-4 minutes per week is reasonable way to get from the 30-minute runs in Phase 1 to 60-minute runs at the end of Phase 2. Be aware that the risk of overuse injuries rises with the time spent running. Squad leaders must weigh the benefit of running greater than 5 miles with the risk of creating lower extremity injuries.

2. Intervals

The purpose of interval training is to build anaerobic endurance and leg power.

Phase 1 - 30/30s

The 30/30 run is named for the run/rest ratio – 30 seconds running pretty hard, 30 seconds walking. The pace for the running should be about 80-90% of your maximum effort, not maximum heart rate. The running portion of the 30/30s should feel like a hard effort that falls short of a full-out sprint. Concentrate on running with good form – head up, shoulders relaxed, trunk directly over the pelvis, arm swing moderate and in line with the direction of travel.

30/30s are the primary form of interval training in phase one and should be performed once per week. In the first few weeks of phase one, perform 10 reps, take a 4-5 minute walking break, then repeat 10 more reps. Add a couple reps to each set during the last weeks of phase one.

Phase 2 & 3 – Track Intervals

Track intervals are a staple of middle and long distance running programs. They are a proven method of improving aerobic and anaerobic fitness and should be included weekly in phases two and three. Use the chart below as a guide to interval training. You may run all intervals at a particular distance or mix in a few of each. Systematically progress the number of intervals over the course of phases two and three. Over the course of phases two and three, you should perform some sessions at each distance.

Distance (meters)	Effort*	# if Intervals	Rest Between Intervals (minutes)
200	90%	15-20	1.5 - 2
400	80%	6-12	1.5 - 3
800	2-mile race pace	3-6	2-3

If a track is not available, base the interval on time:

Time (min:sec)	Effort*	# of Intervals	Rest Between Intervals (minutes)
0:45	90%	15-20	1.5 - 2
1:30	80%	6-12	1.5 - 3
3:00	2-mile race pace	3-6	2-3

*Effort level is used to establish pace. This is a mental calculation taken during the middle portion of the first repetition. The bottom line is to 1) finish the prescribed number of intervals, 2) maintain good running form throughout, 3) have essentially the same time for each interval, and 4) feel that you've challenged yourself.

3. Tempo Run

These runs improve your endurance by increasing your lactic threshold. In effect, you are training your cells to better deal with the natural by-products of running at a relatively high intensity. For our purposes the duration at tempo speed should be about 20 minutes. These runs should be preceded by movement prep and then five minutes of easy jogging. The pace should feel comfortably hard. Basically, you are running just a little below your race pace. So, if you rated a race as 10/10 effort, tempo runs are about an 8/10 effort. If using a heart-rate monitor, stay in the 85-90% of maximum heart rate range. Unless you are training for ½ marathons and beyond, there is no real need to increase the 20-minute duration. Instead, gradually increase the tempo.

4. Fartlek Run

These runs can be used in a variety of ways to build both aerobic and anaerobic endurance. They also should improve your sense of pacing. Fartlek runs are a form of interval training. Periods of faster-paced running are alternated with a slower pace that allows some recovery. Limit these runs to about 30 minutes. Fartleks allow the squad leader maximum flexibility to challenge his Rangers. If available, incorporate hills into the fartlek run by attacking the hill then recovery at the top. Repeats on the same hill are not considered fartlek training, but can occasionally be substituted for fartleks.

Secondary Runs

5. 300-yard Shuttle Run Repeats

This run should be used in conjunction with other non-running workouts. For example, it is a good supplement to a workout from the strength or tactical categories.

Beginning from a crouch start, run three complete round trips between two lines spaced 50 yards apart for a total of 300 yards. Turn by placing at least one foot on or over the line at each turn. Turn to the right for the first change of direction then alternate L/R for the remaining turns. On the final trip, sprint past the Start/Finish Line. Perform repeats with 2-minute recovery breaks between reps. This drill can also be performed over a 25-yard field, using six down-and-backs.

6. Terrain Run

Terrain (cross-country) runs accustom the men to uneven terrain and slopes. This in turn trains the stabilizing muscles of the legs and core that keep the body balanced on uneven terrain. In addition, hill terrain contributes to lower extremity strength/endurance.

Leaders should use these runs judiciously because they carry a higher risk for ankle and knee sprains. Consider the risk during dark or wet conditions. If you choose very rough terrain, it's best to wear boots and keep the duration short. For easier terrain such as a golf course or dirt trail, running shoes and a longer duration are fine. Relatively short terrain runs are a good supplement to workouts from the strength or battle-focus categories.

7. Foot Marching

Purpose: Develop aerobic endurance with load; toughen the feet;

Utilization: Generally twice per month throughout the Foundation and Endurance Phases (Once on even terrain and the other on an uneven terrain).

Execution: In the early Foundation Phase, the footmarch should cover a distance of no greater than 6 miles with the RF1 packing list not to exceed 45 lbs. In the later Foundation Phase and the Endurance Phase, leaders gradually increase the distance and load. Long distance footmarching (15+ miles) should be considered for the development of mental toughness. Such footmarches carry a risk that should be considered and mitigated. The risk for breaking down Rangers can be mitigated by 1) no PT or other high physical demands 1-2 days before and two days after the event, 2) only performing the long marches in the later phases of the program, after core strength has been established, 3) following best practices for foot care and tactical pauses along the march, 3) following good hydration/nutrient replacement practices, 4) ensuring individuals Rangers have had success at the 12-mile distance first.

Power Ruck

Purpose: Improve movement techniques under load while challenging anaerobic power endurance.

Utilization: Used 1-2X/month in Foundation and Endurance Phases. Best used in conjunction with other Tactical PT Drills (Ex. Casualty Evac)

Execution: The assault pack is the preferred load, as it allows for greater speed of movement; however, other load sizes and configurations may be appropriate depending on the goal of the training.

- Climbs

Hills and stairwells are the primary options. When using higher intensity effort (stairwells, short hills), go hard for up to 30-seconds, then rest for twice the length of the work. More moderate intensity efforts (longer hills) can last up to three minutes, followed by rest of an equal duration

- Level Terrain

On level terrain, the increased power demand must come from a heavier pack or faster movement. As mentioned above, the expected mission requirements will dictate pack weight. Work to rest ratios will vary depending on the intensity of the effort. Short, explosive movements such as 3-5 second rushes will require rests periods of at least 2-3X the duration of the rush. Consider using tires, logs, stakes/engineering tape, etc, to set up agility challenges.

- Mixed Terrain

The principles of Fartlek and Terrain runs can be used for an effective power ruck session. As with Fartlek runs, leaders must be in tune with their men's stamina and adjust the speed/load accordingly. Moving back and forth from roads, trails, sand, and grassy fields challenges the body's stabilizers. Seek out rolling terrain to further challenge the stabilizing demand. Save the more challenging mixed-terrain power rucks for phase two and three.

8. Swimming

Purpose: Primarily used as an aerobic workout that provides relative rest for the weight-bearing bones/joints. The principles of interval training can also be applied to swimming or deep-water running (best with an aqua jogger belt) to create an anaerobic workout with little joint stress.

Utilization: Because of the non weight-bearing nature of swimming, it can be performed frequently and is a good choice for a second workout of the day. Leaders should consider swimming as the primary workout of the day on those occasions when the legs need recovery from the previous day's workout or during recovery weeks.

Execution: For aerobic conditioning, swim at a steady pace for 20-60 minutes. For inefficient swimmers that fatigue easily, a combination of swimming and deep-water running with a flotation vest is a good option. For anaerobic conditioning, there are many variations on interval training for runners that can be applied to the pool.

Running Form

Most discussions of how to improve running center around various workouts designed to improve speed. Often overlooked, however, it is the efficiency of running form. Since running form among elite runners can vary significantly, there is a tendency to let the individual find a gait to their liking and leave it alone. Indeed, running is a very fluid, natural act that may be inhibited by over-analysis. However, there are several things runners can do to improve their efficiency without overhauling their natural style. Most runners will find one or two points on which they can improve.

- Head: The head should remain over its base of support – the neck, with the chin neither pointing up or down. Allowing the head to ride forward puts undue strain on the muscles of the upper back.
- Shoulders: The shoulders should assume a neutral posture – neither rounded forward nor forcefully arched backward. Rounding the shoulders forward is the most common fault in everyday posture as well as with running. This is usually associated with tightness of the chest and shoulders. Another problem occurs when the shoulder girdle starts to rise with fatigue or increased effort. This position not only wastes energy, but can also adversely affect breathing.
- Arms: Throughout the arm swing, the elbows should stay at roughly a 90-degree bend. The wrists stay straight and the hands remain loosely cupped. The arm swing should be free of tension, but do not allow the hands to cross the midline of the body.
- Trunk and Pelvis: Like the head, the trunk should remain over its base of support – the pelvis. A common problem with fatigue is allowing the trunk to get in front of the legs and pelvis. This forces the lower back muscles to spend too much energy resisting further trunk collapse to the front.
- Legs: For distance running, much of the power comes from below the knee. Energy is wasted as the knees come higher and the big muscles around the hips and thighs get involved. Practice getting a strong push-off at the ankle joint. This helps to naturally lengthen the stride. Lengthening the stride by reaching forward with the front leg will be counterproductive.
- Feet: For most Rangers, the feet should be pointing directly forward while running. With fatigue, flat feet, and certain muscle imbalances, the legs and feet will start to rotate outward. This hinders performance and may create abnormal stresses that cause injury.

Barefoot/Minimalist Running

Despite several studies being conducted that compare wearing running shoes to no or minimal footwear (i.e. Vibram Five Fingers (VFF), New Balance Minimus, Merrell Trail Gloves, etc.), no research has been able to comprehensively conclude that one type of running is better than the other. Below is a brief list of what current available research indicates:

- Barefoot/minimalist running **might**:
  - Improve or impair running biomechanics (e.g. technique/form)
  - Decrease injury rates in the leg and/or knee
  - Increase injury rates in the thigh, hip, and/or low back
  - Decrease or increase force exerted into the ground through the foot on each impact/stride

Most Rangers are more familiar with what they might have heard from other Rangers or from other media sources (such as other training websites, training programs, and advertisements):

- Barefoot/minimalist running **might**:
  - Increase foot strength
  - Improve arch support
  - Decrease plantar fasciitis issues
  - Increase soft tissue injuries of the foot and ankle
  - Increase OR decrease overall running performance (e.g. speed, duration, etc.)

When considering the research that is currently available as well as abundant and consistent anecdotal self-reports from Rangers, the points below summarize the current guidance from the RAW cell on barefoot/minimalist running.

- If you chose to run barefoot, in VFFs, or any other minimalist footwear:
  - This is not a magical fix to pain experienced due to running. Those who have decreased pain and injury with barefoot/minimalist running appears to achieve this mostly because they were previously a "heel striker" and changed their running style to a mid-foot or forefoot running style. This change in running style is what ultimately decreases the force that the runner exerts into the ground as well as the force that is sent like a shockwave through the body upon each contact of the foot with the ground.

  - Increasing your duration of running without a typical running shoe takes time. Common guidance is to start with no more than 400 meters each day in the first 2-3 weeks. This allows you to toughen your feet and <u>correctly alter your running gait/style</u> to take full advantage of this change in footwear.

  - After the first initial weeks of training, <u>slowly</u> increase volume and include speed work at a rate that is noticeably slower than a normal running program that is based on use of typical running shoes.
    - Any time you change your footwear or running style you need to go back to a walk-to-run progression. This should last as long as needed until you can walk 2 miles in 30 minutes or less in the new footwear, without pain. If you can walk 2 miles in 30 minutes then add running with a 10% increase per week until you achieve the distance and duration desired.

  - For the majority of the Ranger population, barefoot/minimalist running is likely not the best option for running long distances. Though it may be possible to train the entire body to run for long distances in minimal to no footwear, this type of physical development would likely require a training program that is significantly longer than what is now typical (i.e. years rather than months) in order to be done properly.

- Consider the length of time you have spent standing/walking/running in normal (padded) footwear throughout your entire life versus barefoot or in minimal footwear. Your tissues in your body (bones, muscles, tendons, and ligaments) need sufficient time to respond and recover from the new stimuli it's receiving in regards to biomechanics and a newer, unusual type of physical conditioning.

  o When transitioning to barefoot/minimalist training, it may be advisable in a single session to run briefly in minimalist footwear and then switch to regular running shoes (or first in running shoes then briefly in minimalist footwear) so that a planned running session does not have to be cut short and cause a loss of time spent on cardiovascular conditioning.

  o Wearing minimalist footwear during PT sessions that don't require running (e.g. lifting weights, calisthenics, etc.) may help to strengthen your feet and help accelerate the time it takes to train up without injury.

  o Read up on the footwear and make sure that you try it on before you purchase it.

- If you choose NOT to run barefoot or any other minimalist footwear:
  o Padded shoes cannot prevent a poorly designed running program. Running more than 3 times a week (averaging no more than 30 minutes) in any type of footwear significantly increases PT injuries for Rangers.

Goals, training history, and personal preference always play into any decision when it comes to human performance and training. If you have any questions regarding your individual specific needs or goals, follow-up with your strength and conditioning coach or your physical therapist for additional guidance.

Principles of Movement Skills Training

BOTTOM LINE UP FRONT – RAW BULLETS FOR MOVEMENT SKILLS:

- Take time to learn the correct movement. When teaching, do the same. This means planning PT sessions to allow sufficient teaching time. You will have to sacrifice a conditioning effect on those days you teach new drills, but your men will be better in the long run.

- You need to be fresh to master complex change of direction movements. Don't smoke your guys and then expect them to do well in agility/power drills or obstacles.

- Within a given PT session, it's best to place movement skills training right after movement prep. If the schedule dictates agility/power drills after other activities, the men will be somewhat fatigued. In such cases, the squad leader should take a little extra time before beginning agility/power drills and avoid pushing the intensity/duration of the session too hard.

Methodology for RAW Movement Skills Training

Movement skills are what link your strength and endurance to the actual physical task at hand. For example, negotiating obstacles requires not only strength and endurance, but movement skills that make execution of each obstacle safe and efficient.

Movement skills can be grouped into three broad categories: agility, balance, coordination (ABCs). Agility is the ability to change direction, balance is maintaining your center of gravity in an effective position relative to your base of support, and coordination is the ability to effectively do more than one thing at a time. These skills are best developed in childhood, but improvements can be made through training at any age.

In the strength section, we talked about the type of strength Ranger needs. For effective movement skill, strength means control of forces acting on the body. Muscles work either to move or prevent movement at the joints around which they live. Most often we focus on the movement that muscles create because that is what is most apparent. Less obvious though is the "braking" force that muscles apply to joint movement. Without this braking effect, nearly all movement would be extremely sloppy and potentially dangerous.

Around the body's core, this braking action of the trunk muscles becomes extremely important for a couple reasons. First, the spine and pelvis is the base of attachment for many muscles that power the arms and legs. Secondly, the body's center of gravity is within the core area. Keeping it there leads to balanced, skillful movement. This is the job of the core muscles and they do it primarily by putting on the brakes.

For example, in agility training we create drills where momentum is taking the body in one direction, but the task requires change of direction. This requires a level of braking strength, but it also requires awareness of body position. This is very evident during cutting movements. To turn a corner effectively, not only do you need braking strength to slow down your momentum, but you also need an effective movement strategy. Generally, this means lowering the body, planting on the outside leg, and preventing the ankle and knee from rolling outward. You can be strong as an ox, but if your ankle and knee roll to the outside every time you try to cut, you won't be very effective.

These movement strategies must eventually become subconscious. Think of them as your default settings. If your default settings aren't appropriate, your movement will be inefficient. Some degree of conscious awareness of the correct movement, combined with repetitive, controlled drills will usually help. Such drills develop muscle memory, with the goal that the movement quickly becomes automatic – your default setting.

Execution of RAW Movement Skills Training

1. 360-Core

Purpose: Promote core stability and endurance in all planes.

Utilization: This drill should be performed 1-3 times per week in all phases. Development of core stability is a critical component of the RAW program. In Transition Phase #1, the emphasis is on mastering the correct positions and movements, not creating a smoke session. Sloppy execution likely does more harm than good. Once the men have demonstrated solid technique, the advanced techniques can be added and duration of the drill progressed. Per the Physical Training Menu, the Ring of Fire or Med Ball Drills may be substituted for the 360-Core, or two drills may be combined.

Execution:

This drill is performed on the ground, alternating between exercises that work the front, back, and sides of the core. Minimize or eliminate rest between exercises by moving directly to the next position, keeping the core muscles engaged throughout. The plank and bridging exercises are best performed for hold time as opposed to repetitions. Rather than hold for maximum duration, it is best to hold 5-30seconds, then smoothly transition to the next position. The other exercises can be performed for reps or time.

Front Side Emphasis

Plank (Progress to 3-point then 2-point diagonal support)
PU+ with Left and Right Arcs
Supine Bicycle
Double Crunch

R/L Side Emphasis
Side-Bridge (Progress to alternating single leg support)

Back Side Emphasis
Supine Bridge (left leg support)
Supine Bridge (right leg support)
Reverse Plank (Progress to 3-point support)
Prone Row

Plank

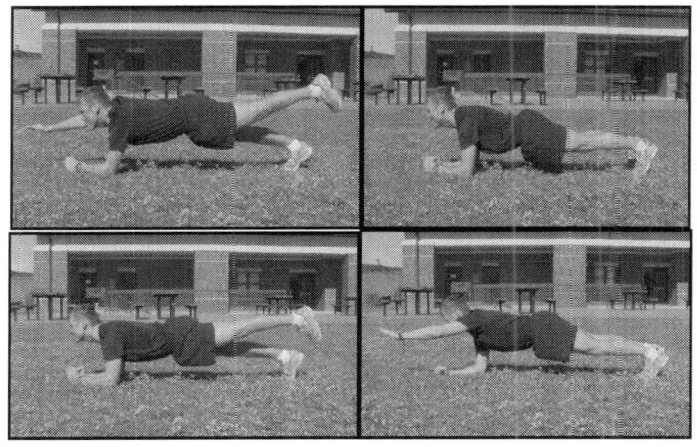

- Maintain rigid alignment of the trunk and legs while supported on the forearms and toes.
- Advance to 3-point support (lift an arm or leg) only if perfect form can be maintained for several 20-second sets.
- Advance to 2-point support (lift opposite arm and leg) only if perfect 3-point support can be maintained for several 20-second sets.
- Look down to keep the head aligned with the trunk…and breathe.

Supine Bridge

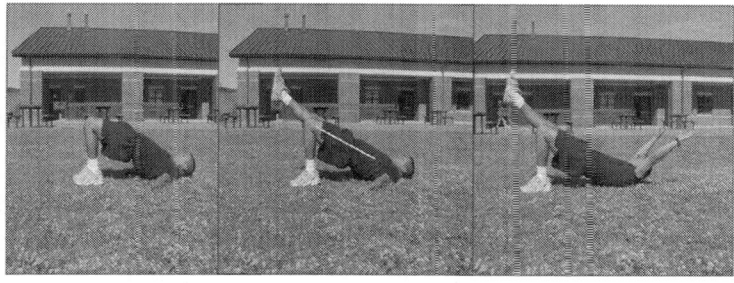

- Raise the hips, supported by the upper back and feet.
- Keep the head off the ground with the chin tucked
- Lift one leg and straighten at the knee. Keep the leg aligned with the trunk. Do not let the pelvis sag down on the side that side.
- Hold 5 seconds, then switch legs without lower the hips. As long as form remains perfect, continue to alternate legs.
- Advanced techniques include arms overhead and/or heels starting farther from the body.

Side Bridge

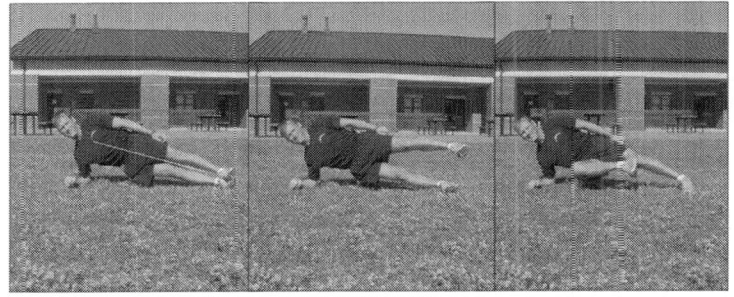

- Support body weight with the forearm and stacked legs, then raise the hips to bring the body into straight alignment.
- Attempt to hold rigidly for 20 seconds. Alternately, perform slow, controlled repetitions for 20 seconds.
- Advanced techniques include bottom or top leg support only. The drill can also be performed with the bottom elbow (right in pictures above) extended and the hand on the ground.

Reverse Plank

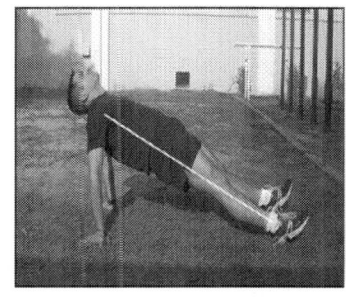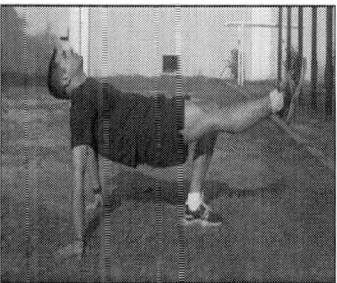

- Support body weight with the arms and feet while maintaining rigid alignment of the trunk and legs. Keep the core muscle tight throughout.
- Don't hyperextend the elbows.
- Attempt to hold for 20 seconds
- Advance to the 3-point position (picture on the right) by flexing the support leg to 90 degrees and lifting the other leg to bring it in line with the trunk.

45

PU+ Left and Right Arc

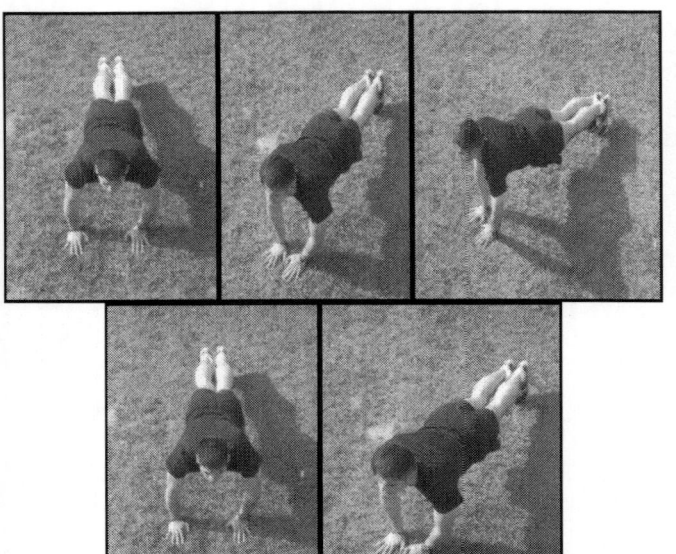

- Begin in the front-leaning-rest position. Perform the push-up plus by pressing with the shoulder blades to raise the chest higher off the ground. Maintain this position throughout the exercise.
- Keeping the feet in place, slowly "walk" with the hands in an arc to the left, return to the middle, repeat to the right.

Double Crunch

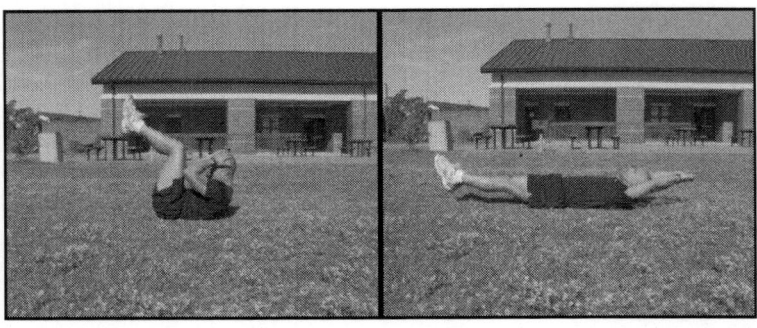

- Perform at a slow pace.
- Attempt to touch the elbows to the knees with the feet off the ground, and then maximally extend the body by reaching with the arms and legs.
- Lower the arms and legs to within a few inches of the ground, but do not allow the low back to arch off the ground.

Prone Row

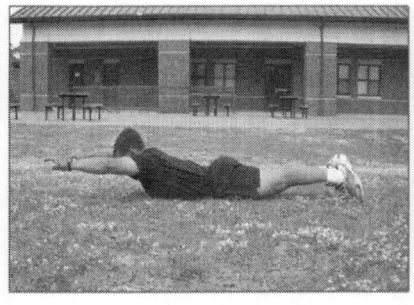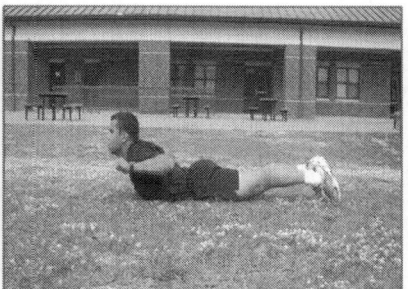

- Begin with the arms overhead a few inches off the ground and the head in line with the rest of the body.
- Slowly lift the head and chest and perform a rowing motion with the arms, keeping the forearms parallel to the ground. The shoulder blades should pinch together.
- Lifting the legs may excessively increase pressure on the lower spine and is not recommended.

Supine Bicycle

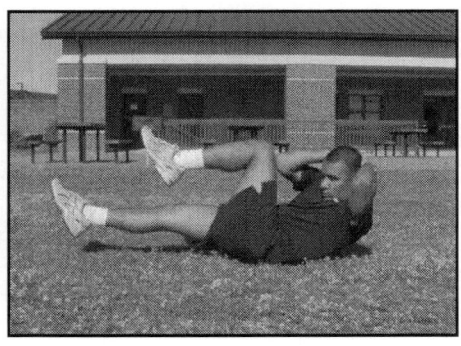

- Perform 1 set for 1 minute.
- Perform at a slow pace without jerking on the neck.
- Attempt to touch the elbow to the opposite knee.
- Reach as far as possible with the straight leg and lower it slowly to within a few inches of the ground.
- Do not allow the low back to arch off the ground.

2. Elastic Band Resistance

Purpose: Promote core stability and endurance in standing. The drill engages the lower extremity and core muscle while demanding teamwork (if performing Ring of Fire) and attention to detail.

Utilization: Can be performed 1-2X/week in all phases. In the Foundation Phase, the emphasis is on mastering the correct positions and movements, not creating a smoke session. Sloppy execution likely does more harm than good. Once the men have demonstrated solid technique, the advanced techniques can be added and duration of the drill progressed.

Execution: Anchor elastic band to any permanent structure. All commands come from the squad/ring leader. Perform each exercise for 1 minute. For example, perform one minute of the Side-Step Squat to the left and one minute to the right. Several repetitions of each exercise can be performed within one minute. Maintain the end position (most tension in the band) for 3-5 seconds. Always maintain body control. For most drills, this means maintaining the power stance.

Safety Note: For the side-step and other lateral movements, always pivot back toward the middle before stepping toward the middle to avoid twisting the knee and ankle.

Basic Movements

Side-Step Squat Left/Right
Backward Walk to Squat
Walking Lunge Away from Circle
Bear Walk
Backward Walk with Side-Step (½ circle in each direction)
Lateral Lunge and Twist L/R (Using Arms)
Backward Walk to Squat and Row (Using arms, first set straight row, second set hand over hand)

Optional Progression
Backward Walk to Single-Leg Support
Forward Walk to Single-Leg Support

Side-Step Squat Left/Right

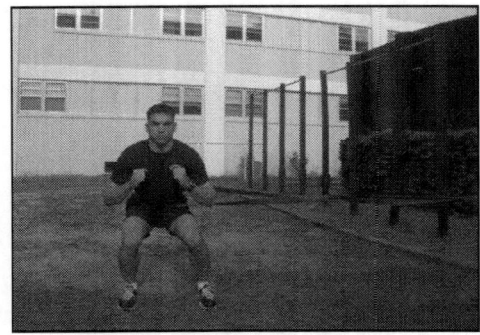

- On the command, "Ready," move into the power stance, facing L or R.
- On the command, "Move," start side stepping away from the ring. Each Ranger coordinates their movement with the group, keeping the ring centered.
- On the command, "Hold," stop moving the feet, squat lower, and hold until the next command.
- On the command, "Recover," rise out of the squat and at the same time pivot toward the ring. Slowly walk back toward the ring, but do not allow the ring to touch the ground.

Walking Lunge Away

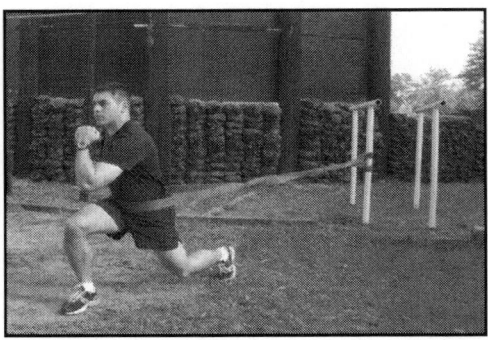

- On the command, "Ready," move into the power stance crouch, facing away from the ring.
- On the command, "Move," begin taking lunge steps away from the ring. Each Ranger coordinates their movement with the group, keeping the ring centered.
- On the command, "Hold," stop stepping, lower into a full lunge, and hold until the next command.
- On the command, "Recover," rise slowly out of the lunge and return toward the ring taking controlled rear lunge steps. Do not allow the ring to touch the ground.

Backward Walk to Squat

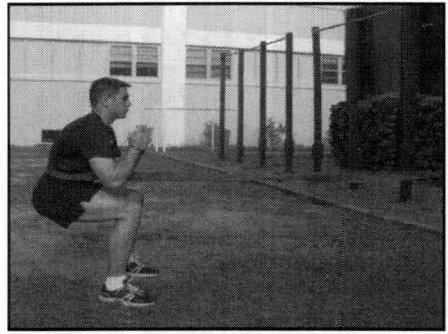

- On the command, "Ready," move into the power stance, facing the ring.
- On the command, "Move," back-peddling away from the ring. Each Ranger coordinates their movement with the group, keeping the ring centered.
- On the command, "Hold," stop moving the feet, squat lower, and hold until the next command.
- On the command, "Recover," rise out of the squat and slowly walk back toward the ring. Do not allow the ring to touch the ground.

Bear Walk

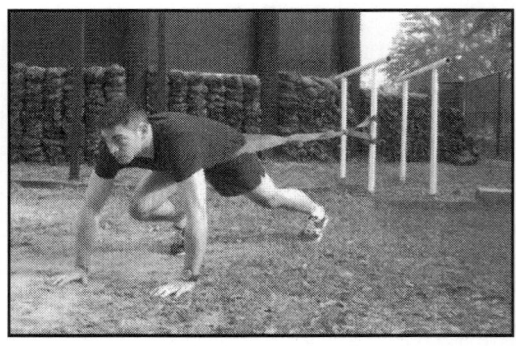

- On the command, "Ready," move into mountain climber position, facing away from the mount.
- On the command, "Move," begin bear walk steps away from the mount.
- On the command, "Hold," stop moving and hold that position until the next command.
- On the command, "Recover," _remain on all fours_ and slowly bear walk in.

Backward Walk with Side-Step

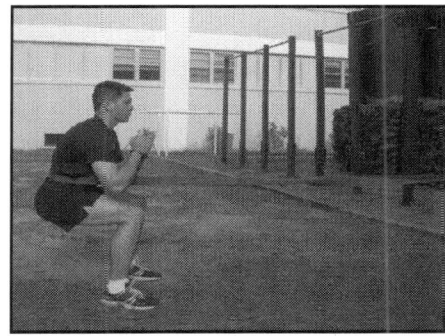

- Begin as per the Backward Walk to Squat. Once holding in that position, the next command is, "Move Left."
- Begin taking side-steps to the left. Maintain full tension in the band.
- On the command, "Hold," stop moving the feet, squat lower, and hold until the next command.
- On the command, "Move Right," begin taking side-steps to the right.
- On the command, "Hold," stop moving the feet, squat lower, and hold for 3-5 seconds.

Backward Walk to Squat and Double Row

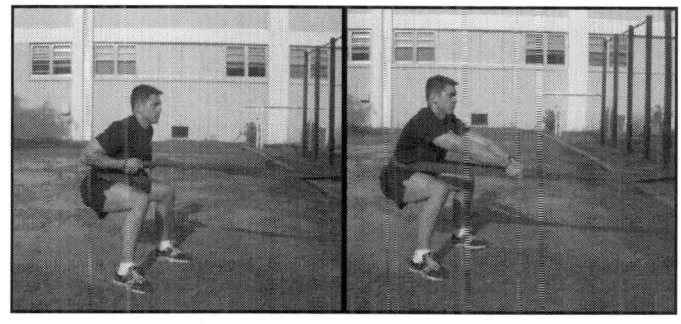

- First, perform the Backward Walk to Squat per the previous guidance.
- Next, use the "Pull/Recover" commands to perform 8-10 reps of the row (shown above).

Lateral Lunge and Twist Left/Right

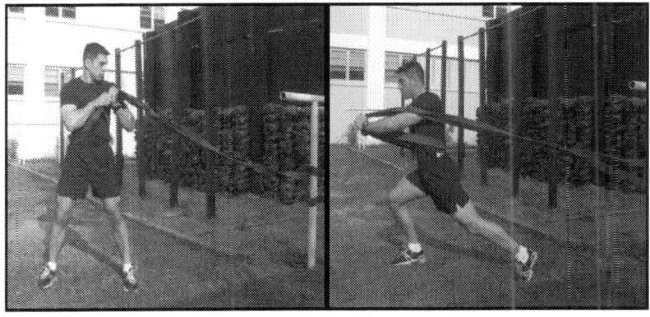

- Face left or right, with some slack in the band.
- On the command, "Ready," grab the band with a two-hand grip.
- On the command, "Pull," pull the band across the body while taking a lunge step away from the ring. (No hold command needed.)
- On the command, "Recover," return to the starting position.
- Repeat the "Pull/Recover" for 8-10 reps, and then switch directions.

Backward Walk to Squat and Single Row

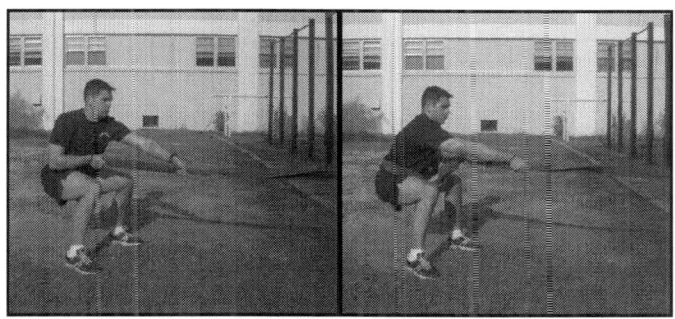

- First, perform the Backward Walk to Squat per the previous guidance.
- Next, use the "Pull/Recover" commands to perform 8-10 reps of the row using the hand-over-hand technique shown above.

MedBall Drills (Core Stability Emphasis)

Purpose: Develop core stability for both short and long-range explosive movements; provides resistance to movement in all planes.

Utilization: Once or twice per week in all phases. The session lasts 20 minutes.

Execution: A solid wall is needed for this drill. With one partner working and the other(s) monitoring form, perform the short and medium-range wall-based exercises for 20 seconds, and then switch (40 seconds rest). Progress to 30-second sets, using a 1:1 work-to-rest ratio. The rest time may be progressively reduced. Perform short-range drills in order (2 sets) before the medium-range drills. The short-range drill is meant to be performed at maximal intensity. The first couple throws are used to get the rhythm, but then it is balls to the wall intensity.

For the partner, medium-range drills, the intensity should be reduced and each exercise maintained for 1 minute. Rest briefly (about 10 seconds) before the next exercise in the drill.

Ensure core stability throughout the work phase. If fatigue causes improper technique, stop no matter the time on the clock. Choose a medball weight that allows completion of the drill.

Short-Range (against wall, 2 sets)
    Chest Toss
    Overhead Toss
    Overhead Toss Staggered-Stance Left
    Overhead Toss Staggered-Stance Right
    Rotation Toss Left
    Rotation Toss Right
Medium-Range (against wall, 1 set)
    Chest Toss
    Rotational Toss Left
    Rotational Toss Right
Partner, Medium-Range (1 min each)
    Underhand Toss
    Rotational Toss L
    Rotation Toss R
Optional Substitutions
    Underhand Diagonal (wall)
    Backward Over-the-Shoulder (wall)

Chest Toss Short-Range

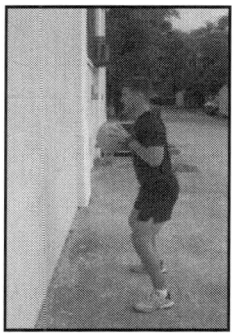

- Remain in the power stance with core muscles tight throughout the drill.
- Bounce the ball vigorously off the wall and catch at chest height with the ball just a few inches away from the chest.
- The first couple throws are relatively slow to ensure proper technique, and then go rapid fire with good form.

Overhead Toss Short-Range

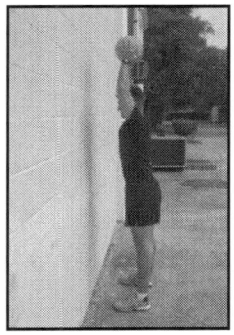

- Keep the core muscles tight throughout the drill. This will prevent the back from arching.
- Bounce the ball vigorously off the wall and catch in the overhead position with the elbows bent.
- The first couple throws are relatively slow to ensure proper technique, and then go rapid fire with good form.

Overhead Toss Staggered L/R Short-Range

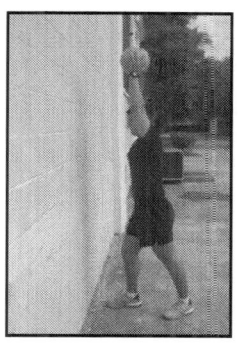

- This drill is the same as the Overhead Toss, except the stance is staggered. Either switch left and right during a set or perform an equal number of left and right sets. Keep the core muscles tight throughout the drill. This will prevent the back from arching.
- Bounce the ball vigorously off the wall and catch in the overhead position with the elbows slightly bent.
- The first couple throws are relatively slow to ensure proper technique, and then go rapid fire with good form.

Rotation Toss L/R Short-Range

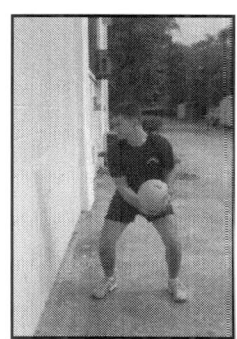

- Remain in the power stance with core muscles tight throughout the drill.
- Use a scooping motion of the arms to throw the ball vigorously off the wall. The arms perform most of the work, with the trunk rotating slightly with each toss.
- Do not let the ball rebound beyond the point shown in the picture.
- The first couple throws are relatively slow to ensure proper technique, and then go rapid fire with good form.

Chest Toss Medium-Range

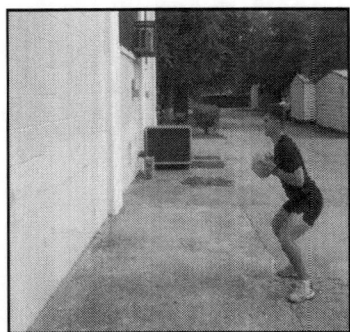

- This drill is a slower, but more explosive version of the short-range Chest Toss.
- Stand 5-6 feet from the wall, crouch into the power stance with the ball at the chest, and then explode out of that stance to throw the ball.
- Throw the ball hard enough so that it hits the wall at about head level.
- The ball should be caught at chest level, with the body back in the power stance.
- Although the legs flex and extend, the feet should remain in place.
- Emphasis is on explosive/powerful movement and maintaining good form

Rotation Toss L/R Medium-Range

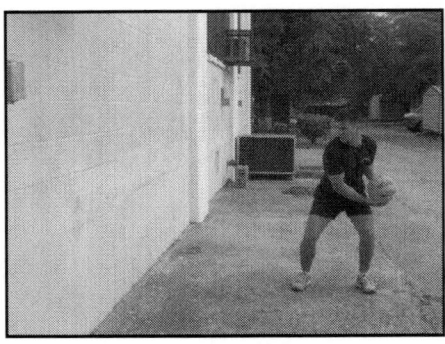

- This drill is a slower, but more explosive version of the short-range Rotation Toss.
- Stand 5-6 feet from the wall in the power stance with the ball held outside the leg farthest from the wall. Most of the body weight should be on the outside leg. Rise explosively out of the power stance and whip the ball to the wall, transferring weight to the inside leg.
- Throw the ball hard enough that it hits the wall at about shoulder height and returns.
- The catch should end back in the starting position.

3. Speed/Agility/Coordination Drills

The purpose of this drill is to optimize movement skills and improve reaction, speed, and change-of-direction.

A. Speed/Quickness Drills

Always perform the speed prep drill first: 1 rep over a 10-20M segment.
For the speed/quickness drill, perform 2 or 3 progressive repetitions (don't start out at 100%). The distance for each repetition should be about 20-40 yards. Walk slowly back to the start point. This should not be a highly fatiguing drill in **Phase 1**, when the work-to-rest ratio should be about 1:5. In **Phase 2**, the rest time can be decreased, though form should never be compromised during these drills. Attempting to sprint through fatigue will only promote injury. Do not race – instead concentrate on form.
Performance Note: For the Athletic Stance Lateral Sprint, the first movement consists of simultaneously bringing the lead leg back under the body's center of gravity (rather than stepping) and pivoting the trail leg to line up the body in the direction of travel.

Speed Prep
Butt-Kick Walk
High-Knee Walk
Butt Kick Jog
Walking Forward Leg Kicks (Ballistic Hamstring Stretch)
Verticals

Speed/Quickness Drill
Verticals to Sprint
Forward Falls to Sprint (with partner, without, then partner breakaways)*
Mountain Climber to Sprint
Athletic Stance to Lateral Sprint (10 meters only)

*Forward Falls are a foundational drill best used in **Phase 1**. In **Phase 2**, use only the partner breakaways.

Agility/Coordination Drills

It is best to begin with the speed skater, which is performed in place. The next two preliminary drills should begin at a modest intensity (the "sprint" should be a 70-80% effort). The other drills are performed to the distances indicated. As with all skill training drills, group leaders should observe for sloppy movement due to fatigue or lack of concentration. Especially in **Phase 1**, emphasis should be on correct execution, not creating a smoke session. Also be aware of field conditions and adjust speed of movement as necessary to avoid slips and falls.

The drills can be used to create a circuit, spending about 2 minutes each at the ladder, cones and low hurdle stations, with a fourth station chosen from among the other drills listed below.

Preliminary Drills
-Speed Skater (8-10 progressive reps in each direction as agility prep)

-Laterals to Run (10-20 yards of laterals then 10-20 yard sprint)
-Crossover to Run (10-20 yards of crossovers, then 10-20 yard sprint)
-Run and Reach (20-40 yards moving forward; reaching every third step)

Agility Ladder
    -Forward Shuffle (May substitute forward run - each foot in each square)
    -Lateral Shuffle

Cones (8-10 cones, 3 ft apart)
    -Forward Shuffle
    -Lateral Shuffle (stagger the cones)

Low Hurdles (8-10 hurdles, 2-3 ft apart)
    -Lateral Step-Over
    -Forward High Step

Cuts – (4 cones or other markers placed 10 yards apart)
    -45-degree cuts
    -90-Degree Cuts
    -Triangles (10 yards apart; alternate R/L direction)

Other Agility Options
    -Lateral Shuffle Reaction Drill (performed on the squad leader's command over a 5-15 meter area in each direction (do not pause when changing direction)
    -Drop Step Shuffle (40-yard length; change direction every 5 yards)
    -3-5 second rushes
    -T-Drill (10 yards for each segment of the "T")
    -Illinois Agility Test

Butt-Kicks Walk/Jog

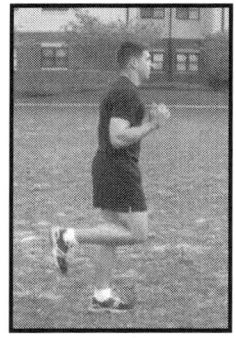

- Begin at walking speed
- Fire the hamstrings to lift the heel quickly to the butt.
- Do not let the knee go forward of the trunk.
- When the left leg is on the ground, the right arm is forward.
- After a few kicks with each leg, break into an easy-pace jog using the same technique.
- Perform over a 20-30 yard segment.

Walking Forward Leg Kicks

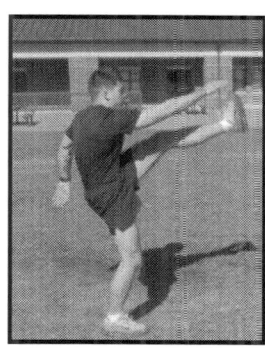

- This drill is similar to the high knee walk, but adds a quick kick to straighten the leg and stretch the hamstring.
- Maintain a tall stance. Do not lean forward at the trunk.
- Keep the intensity and range of motion relatively low for the first few kicks, then gradually kick faster and farther.
- The height of the kick will vary greatly among the men due to difference in hamstring length. Do not attempt to have everyone kick to the same height.
- Perform over a 10-20 yard segment.

High Knee Walk

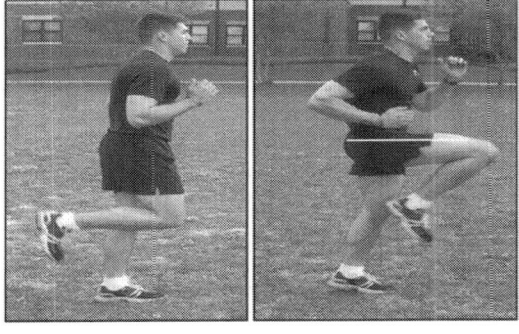

- This drill combines the butt-kick walk with a high step. It improves running efficiency, especially for sprints.
- Immediately after performing the butt-kick, lift the knee quickly to the front to hip level.
- Use strong arm action as shown in the pictures.
- Perform over a 20-30 yard segment.

Verticals to Sprint

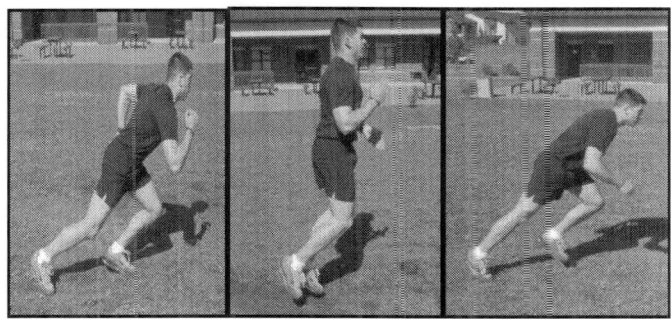

- Perform verticals as per the movement prep guidance.
- At the 10 yard mark, transition into a sprint by leaning the entire body forward over the next few strides. Do not bend forward at the waist to transition to a sprint. Continue to use strong arm action and a tall stance once you hit the sprint stride.

Forward Fall to Sprint

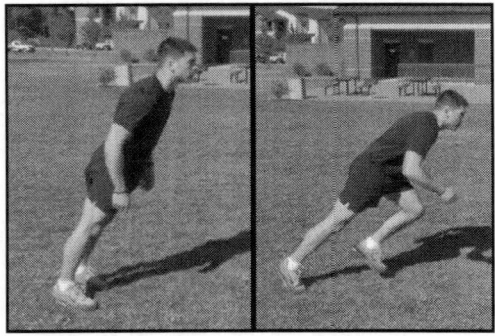

- Next perform 3-4 forward falls unassisted. Without a partner to catch you, fire out into a 15-20 yard sprint. Do not pause after the first step, but rather use the forward momentum of the body to "roll" into a sprint.

Forward Falls-Partner Resisted

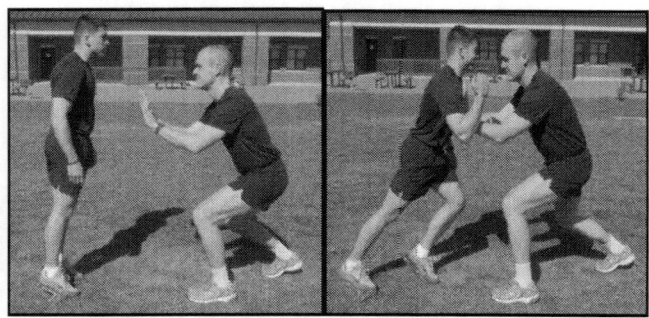

- Begin with partner falls. The "sprinter" rises onto the toes, then lets the body fall forward while keeping straight alignment from head to toe. The partner catches the sprinter at the collar bone and upper chest as the sprinter performs one very quick but short first step. The sprinter's arms fire quickly into the sprint ready position. Perform 3-4 reps on each leg. The two keys to this drill are 1) letting the straight body fall forward maximally before stepping, and 2) ensuring that the first step is not so long that the foot gets forward of the body's center of gravity.
- Forward Falls are a foundational drill best used in **Phase 1**. In **Phase 2**, use only the partner breakaways.

Partner Breakaways

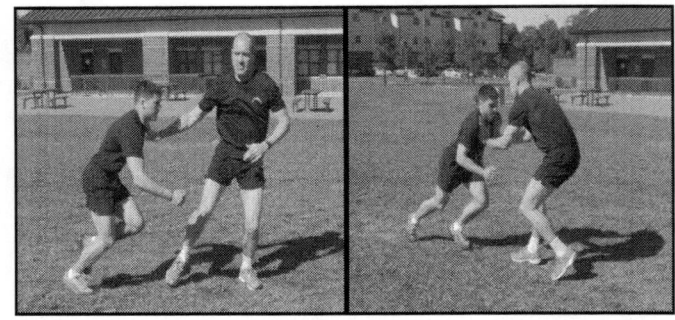

- Perform forward fall with partner as previously described, except add resisted sprint and breakaways-
- The partner provides moderate resistance to the sprinter while back peddling. At about 5-10 yards, The partner turns and releases to sprint alongside the sprinter.
- Forward Falls are a foundational drill best used in **Phase 1**.
- In **Phase 2**, use only the partner breakaways.

Mountain Climber Sprint

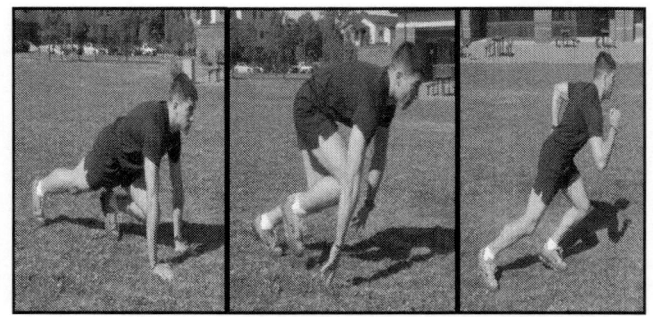

- On the fourth count of the mountain climber exercise, push vigorously from the arms and legs to rise into a sprint.
- Do not pause before rising, but rather use the spring effect of the mountain climber rep to move quickly into the sprint.
- Alternate which leg is forward to begin the exercise, performing an equal number on each leg.

Athletic Stance to Lateral Sprint

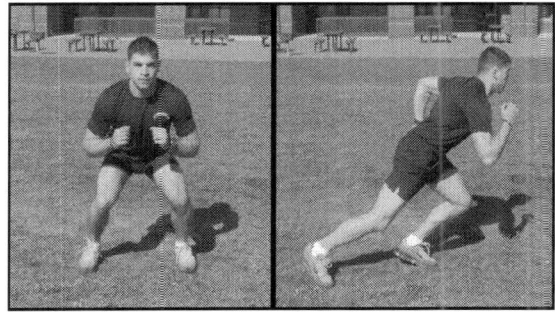

- Start in the athletic/power stance. Let the body drop slightly as you take weight off the legs and perform a pivot in the direction of the lateral sprint.
- The foot of the lead leg should not step out in the direction of the sprint, but should actually be pulled slightly back under the body. This allows the body's center of gravity to get in front of the base of support (lead foot), which in turn gets your momentum going in the direction of the sprint.
- Use strong arm action. During the initial movement, the trailing arm powerfully drives across the body in the direction of the sprint.
- Perform and equal number of sprints in each direction.

Laterals to Run

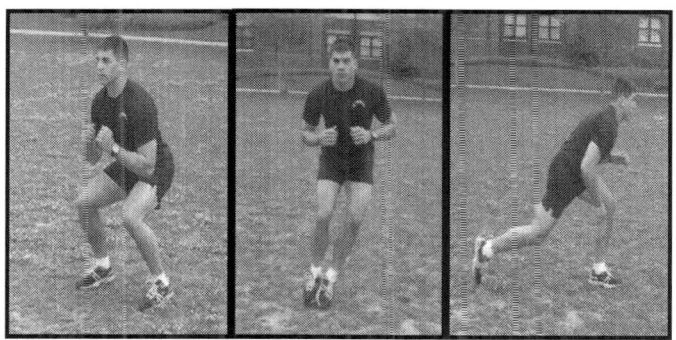

- Perform 10-20 yards of crossovers per the movement prep guidance, then turn and sprint 10-20 yards.
- The lead foot may be turned in the direction of travel or kept parallel to the other foot.
- Perform an equal number of reps in each direction.

Speed Skater

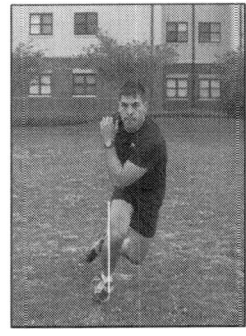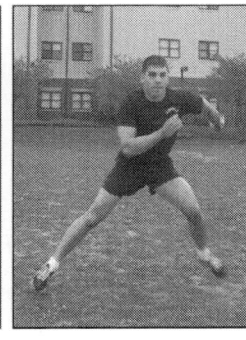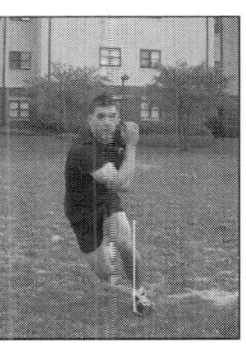

- First step side to side, then add the hop as shown in the middle picture.
- Do not allow momentum to force the knee outside of the foot.
- Do not allow the foot/ankle to roll to the outside – keep the inner edge of the foot firmly in contact with the ground.
- Perform 8-10 progressive reps in each direction.

Crossover to Run

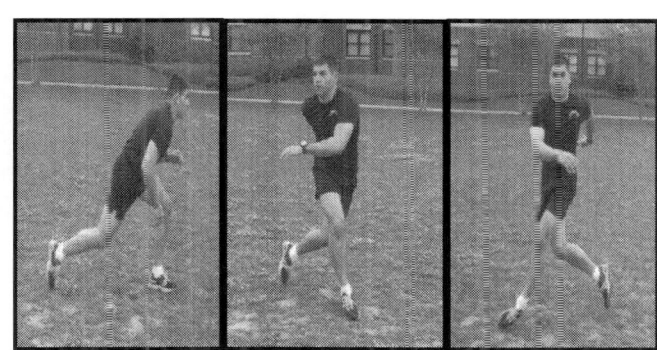

- Perform 10-20 yards of crossovers per the movement prep guidance, then turn and sprint 10-20 yards.
- The lead foot may be turned in the direction of travel or kept parallel to the other foot.
- Perform an equal number of reps in each direction.

Run and Reach

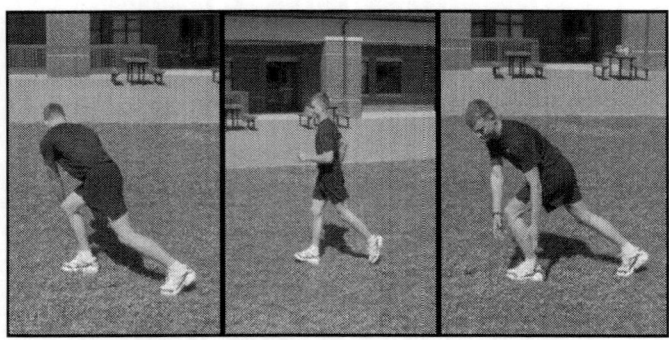

- Perform over 20-40 yards, jogging forward and reaching down and to the outside of the forward leg every third step.
- The first few reps are performed at a modest intensity and range of motion. Gradually increase the speed and range of motion.

Lateral Shuffle (Agility Ladder)

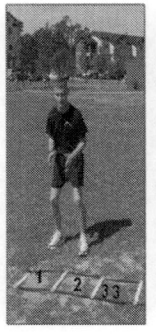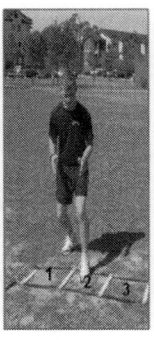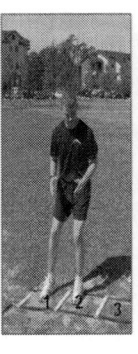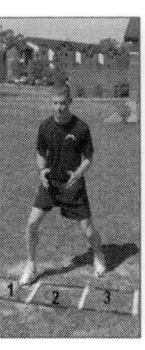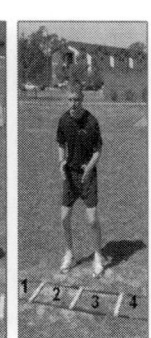

- Step into the second square with the lead (left in picture) foot, then the first square with the trail (right) foot.
- Step out with the lead foot first, then the trail foot.
- When stepping out with the lead foot, place it behind the third square rather than directly behind the second square.
- Step into square four with the lead foot, then square three with the trail foot. Continue down the ladder
- Cadence should be "in, in, out, out" with the lead foot touching in every "even numbered" square and the trail foot in every "odd numbered" square
- Perform an equal number of reps in both directions.

Forward Shuffle (Agility Ladder)

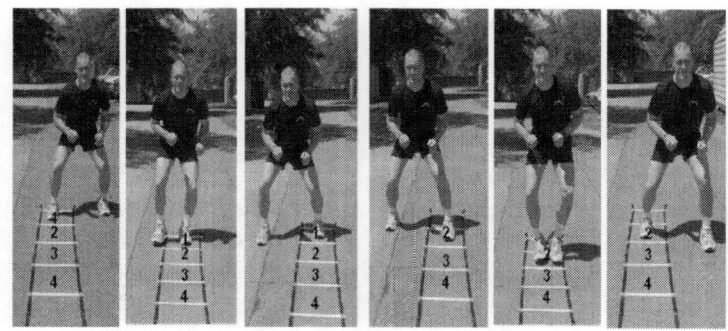

- Crouch with the right foot in the first square.
- Rise out of the crouch and take a shuffle step to the right, so that the left foot is now in the first square.
- Quickly step forward with the left foot into the second square.
- Rise out of the crouch and take a shuffle step to the left, so that the right foot is now in the second square.
- Quickly step forward with the right foot into the third square (not shown), and continue down the ladder.

Forward Shuffle (Cones)

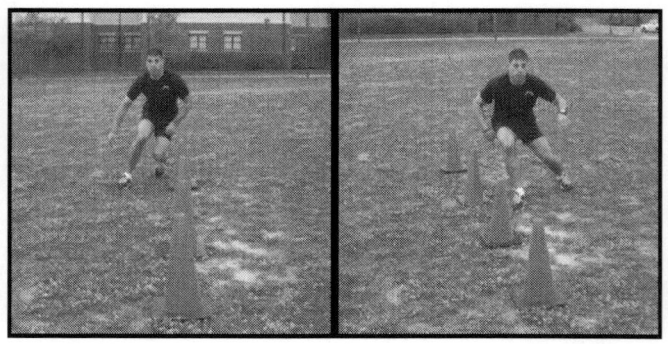

- Running forward through cones spaced about 1 yard apart, plant on the outside leg with plenty of bend in the hip and knee.
- Take a shuffle step between cones, again planting on the outside leg and crouching low.
- Do not allow momentum to force the knee outside of the foot.

Lateral Shuffle (Cones)

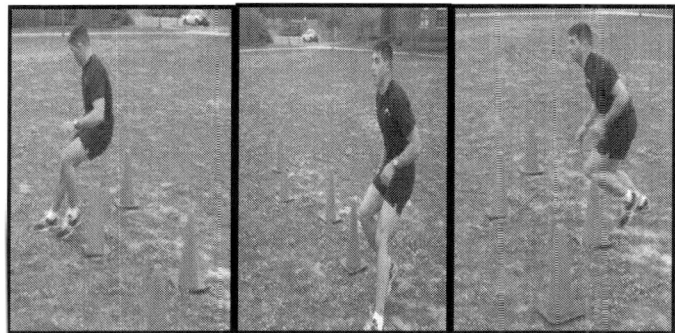

- Stagger the cones and move laterally around the cones, keeping the feet and body directed forward.
- Take short stride, stay in a crouch and control forward/rearward momentum.
- Repeat an equal number of reps in both directions.

Forward High Step (Low Hurdles)

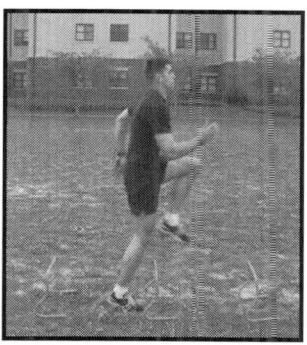

- Stay on the toes and use strong arm action to move over the hurdles.
- Each foot should touch down between each set of hurdles.

Lateral Step-Over (Low Hurdles)

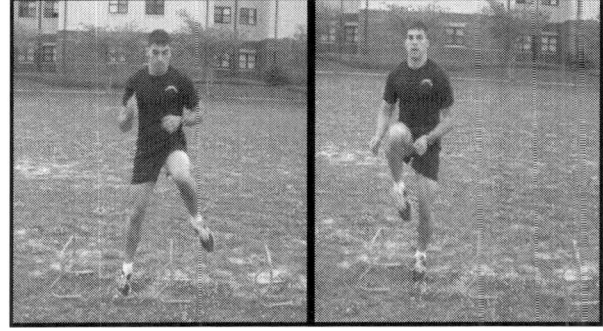

- Stay on the toes and use strong arm action to move over the hurdles.
- Each foot should touch down between each set of hurdles.
- Repeat an equal number of reps in both directions.

Cuts/3-5 Second Rushes

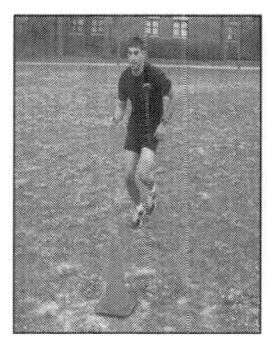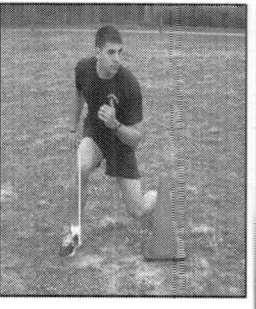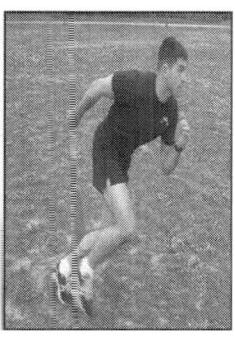

- Space the cones to allow for 3-5 second rushes. Place the cones to allow 45-90 degree cuts
- Sprint to the first cone and do one of the following:
    - Plant and cut to the next cone, ensuring that the outside knee does not drift to the outside of the base of support.
    - Take a knee, pause, then move out to the next cone
    - Go to the prone position, pause, then move out to the next cone

Lateral Step Reaction Drill

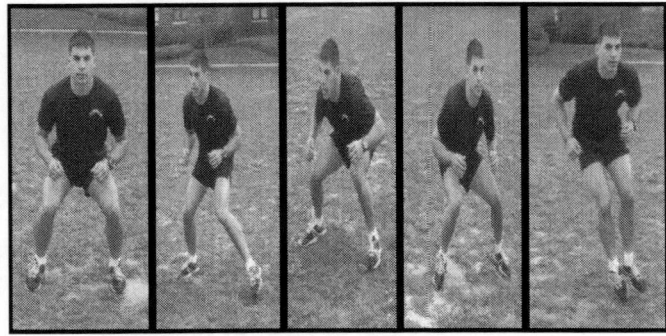

- Include an equal amount of left and right movement. Vary the length of each segment to keep the men guessing as to when the next change of direction will occur.
- Get low at the point of change of direction. Do not allow the foot/ankle to roll to the outside – keep the inner edge of the foot firmly in contact with the ground.
- Do not allow momentum to force the knee outside of the foot.

Drop-Step Shuffle

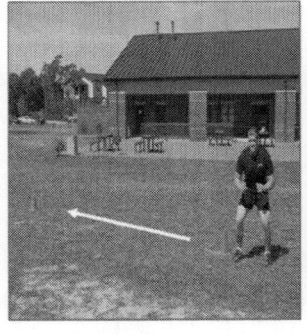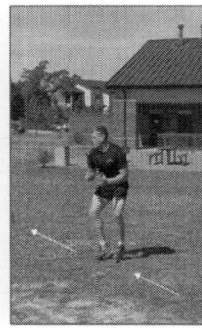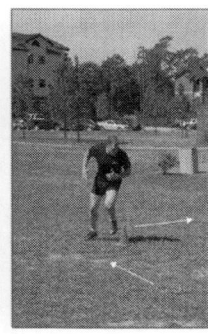

- Angle the body 45 degrees to the right while looking forward.
- Take shuffle steps to the right at a 45 degree angle to the rear.
- After 5 yards, take a quick hop and spin the body around to land in the mirror image position.
- Continue shuffling and changing direction with the hop/spin method for about 40 yards.
- Do not plant and twist the leg to change direction.
- A partner can be used to act as an "offensive player" (running forward and cutting), while the

other RGR reacts to the cuts with the drop step shuffles.

T-Drill

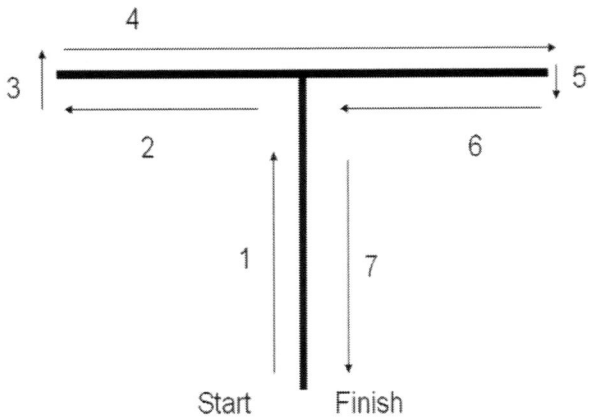

1. Run forward.
2. Crouch and side-step (laterals) to the left.
3. Step forward to move to the other side of the top of the T.
4. Stay in a crouch and side-step to the right.
5. Step backwards to move to the inside of the T.
6. Crouch and side-step (laterals) to the left.
7. Run backwards through the finish line.

Incorporating Hybrid Workouts into RAW

Hybrid workouts blend strength/power and endurance challenges into a single session. There are several advantages to these workouts:

- Efficiency: Time is often in short supply…blended workouts kill two birds with one stone.
- Developing power-endurance: Too many easy-paced long runs will rob the legs of power. When the same endurance effect can be achieve without compromising leg power, the choice is clear. This is not to say we should never run long, only that we should not over-emphasize that mode of training.
- Mental toughness: Most hybrid workouts we've done have required a lot of focus to maintain form as fatigue sets in. Contrast that with mindlessly drifting through a 5-mile run or performing well-rested sets in the weight room.
- Neuro-endocrine response: This basically means nerves and hormones are stimulated. Blending strength and endurance means you are pushing/pulling/lifting something when you are tired. This is hard work and a big stress to the entire body. The body responds by mobilizing a neural and chemical response that gets you better prepared for the next smoke session. This is good, but it requires adequate recovery.

Hybrid workouts have some drawbacks:
- Injury risk: There is nothing inherently risky about hybrid workouts. The risk comes when you choose lifts/exercises for which you are not technically proficient, or you allow form to get sloppy due to fatigue. Unfortunately, we see quite a bit of each risk factor.
- Strength/Power compromise: The restriction on rest intervals compromises strength/power development. Insufficient rest intervals fail to restore creatine-phosphate levels and normal acid-base balances. Rangers wanting to get bigger, stronger, or more powerful must get adequate recovery between sets and, therefore, should limit the use of workouts that don't allow such recovery.
- Over-stimulation of the neuro-endocrine response: This is all about stimulus and response. If you train too hard, too long, you are creating a stimulus to which your body cannot properly respond. Your body will adapt, just not in the way you want (lethargy, low-motivation, higher resting heart rate, immune-suppression, etc.)

Our recommendation for incorporating hybrid workouts is to first define your objectives (both long-term and short-term) and then choose training modes accordingly. Most top athletes follow a periodized approach to training, changing their focus/workouts every few weeks, with a different objective for each period. The classic model trains hypertrophy, strength, power, and sport-specific needs in that order. In this model, hybrid power-endurance workouts fit best during the sport-specific (think Ranger missions) phase. More recently, an alternative training model called non-linear periodization has proven effective. In this model, different forms of strength training are scheduled within a 1-2 week period. Based on discussions with top strength and conditioning researchers, the RAW program recommends this method and includes one heavy-resistance workout, one power-endurance workout, and one local muscle endurance workout per 7-10 day period. The power-endurance workout can be either Ground Base, hybrid, or a combination of the two.

The hybrid, power-endurance workouts certainly have value for Rangers, but should be used as one modality in a broad-ranging PT program rather than the primary mode of training across phases.

Bottom Line Bullets:
- Perform hybrid workouts 1-2X/week in the all phases except Transition #1.
- Lay a good movement skill foundation first.

- o   Understand and control the neutral position of the spine
- o   Perfect form with body-weight squats before heavy squatting, deadlifting, or plyometrics.
- o   Score a "3" on the FMS Deep Squat before weighted, overhead lifts

- Build volume over time. If you have not been training an exercise (Ex: box jumps, kipping pull-ups, handstand pushups), don't do 50, high-speed reps the first session – doing so is a recipe for tendinitis or joint injury.
- Don't let fatigue win…maintain form in the face of deep fatigue. Concentrate!
- Definitely don't let fatigue win with a weight over your head.
- Structure workouts so that more demanding/complex movements (example: Get Ups) are performed early in the workout…before deep fatigue.

Hybrid Drills

1. **Tabata Intervals (Described previously in the Strength chapter)**

2. **Stamina Drill**: Stamina can be defined as the capability of sustaining long, stressful effort. It also means staying power.

Purpose: Challenge multiple energy pathways, local muscle endurance, and willingness to fight through fatigue – this is meant to be an exhaustive drill.

Utilization: Due to the overall intensity of the drill, Rangers must first establish a moderate to high level of endurance and mastery of the component tasks (PU, pull-ups, lunges, etc) before performing the sequence listed below. If using the phased approach, it is best saved for late Foundation Phase or Endurance Phase.

Execution: The order shown below (2-10) represents a basic sequence that can be used for any number of drills with a similar intent. Alternating upper body, lower body, core, and anaerobic running keeps the cardio-respiratory demand high without exhausting any one movement pattern. For variety or preference, one or more of the upper body, lower body, and core sequences can be replaced by combined movements such max-height med ball throws, kettle-bell exercises, tire-flips, etc.

1. Run 8-10 minutes at an easy-moderate pace
2. Alternating sets of push-ups and pull-ups/chin-ups/heel claps: 3 sets each; perform as many perfect repetitions as you can, then switch from pushing to pulling and vice versa; take only 10-20 seconds between sets.
3. Lunge Drill: 2 sets of 20 reps on each leg. Within a given set, perform a variety of lunges (forward, rear, diagonal, side, or transitional lunges)
4. Core Work: One to two minutes using a variety of core exercises (medball slams/wall tosses, 360-core, sit-ups).
5. 300-yard shuttle at a challenging pace (80% effort). Take a two-minute walking recovery (hydrate), then repeat.
6. Repeat PU, pull-up/chin-up/heel clap sets x2
7. Repeat Lunge Drill (15 reps each leg)
8. Repeat Core Work
9. Repeat 300-yard shuttle
10. Repeat the muscular endurance drills (PU, pull-ups/chin-ups/heel claps, lunges, core) x1.
11. Run 8-10 minutes at an easy-moderate pace.

Other options: Tire flips or sled drags in place of 300-yard shuttles; row/bike instead of run.

3. **MedBall Relays**

Purpose: Develop total-body power, agility, and coordination while challenging anaerobic endurance.

Utilization: Rangers must first establish a moderate to high level of endurance and mastery of the component tasks (ex. agility training, med ball throws). These drills are best saved for later phases of training.

Execution: See individual drills below:

One-Bounce MedBall Drill

Perform this drill over a large, flat field of about 100-yard length. One Ranger performs a maximal medicine ball (3 or 4kg) throw (backward/overhead), then races forward past his partner to prepare to receive the partner's throw. The partner race ahead to catch the ball on one bounce, then performs the throw. One partner must catch the MedBall past the 100-yard line and both partners must run to the line. After one catch past the 100-yard line, immediately return in the opposite direction. Attempt to catch the ball from the power stance – do not let momentum from running carry you more than one step past the point where the ball is caught. If the ball is dropped or takes more than one bounce, both partners are penalized (squad leader discretion - 10 seconds added at end or 10 pushups where the ball was dropped).

Suicide Relays
Carry the MedBall while performing suicides over 5, 10, and 20 yards (same course as Partner Shuttle Drill). Touch the MedBall to each line. End the 20-yard segment by running through the Start/Finish line, while handing the ball to the partner. Perform 5 reps, then rest 3-5 minutes and repeat.

Sand Pit Relays
For this variation, start at one end of a sand pit (size of a beach volleyball court). Run to the other end and back (ducking under the net if one is in place), handing the MedBall off to the partner. Perform 5-10 reps then rest and repeat.

4. Partner Shuttle

Purpose: Develop local muscle endurance through calisthenics while challenging anaerobic endurance.

Utilization: May be used in all phases as a time-efficient, field-expedient method for training both strength and endurance. It works well as one of three events on days when the Ground Base circuit is performed by the company.

Execution: One partner runs the shuttle course (down and back over 10, 20, and 30-meter segments) while the other performs calisthenics (PU, SU, supine bicycle, pull-ups, etc.) from the muscular endurance session. If fatigue precludes good form, discontinue calisthenics and begin walking for recovery between shuttle runs. This activity is meant to be performed at high level of intensity. Length of the session is variable based on fitness and the other PT events preceding or following. Generally we start with 6-8 minutes and progress over the phases to longer sessions and/or the addition of kit.

Not a Recovery Day (aka, NARD, pronounced like a pirate)

Get-Ups
One set of 8-12 reps with each arm. Choose a weight that you can control. Alternate sides or perform left and right side sets separately. The kettle-bell is the preferred implement, but dumbbells can work also. Go straight to the next station.

Ground Base Combo Twist
Three timed sets each side (30s, 25s, 20s). Take no rest between sides and minimal time between sets. Load a weight that allows you to maintain speed of movement. Take a short break before moving the next station.

Kettle-Bell Swings
Three sets of 15 reps, choosing the weight accordingly. Rest no more than 30s between sets. Take a short water break as you transition to the next station.

MedBall Throws
We prefer the rotational throws, either with the bouncing MedBall against a wall or the Dynamax balls with a partner. Perform three, 1-minute sets (switching sides at the 30s mark), with no more than a 30s rest between sets. Take a short break before moving the next station.

Air Squat/Push-ups/Pull-ups
Start the clock; perform 15 air squats, 10 push-ups, 5 pull-ups for speed. Rest until the clock strikes 1minute. Continue for 15 minutes. Take a short water break as you transition to the next station.

Anaerobic Big Finish
Row, bike, or sprint for up to three minutes. Consider racing on the rower for 500 meters or track/street for ½ mile.

Purpose: This workout was designed with the core in mind. It also presents a full-spectrum (aerobic and anaerobic) endurance challenge.

Utilization: This is meant to be a stand-along workout, lasting about 45 minutes. Consider doing it once a week for 3-4 weeks, increasing the volume along the way.

Precautions: The first four components of this workout require mastery of technique, especially the Turkish Get-Up. Take the time to master each one separately before combining them into this smoke session. Perform movement prep before this workout.

Notes:

- Perform the Get-Ups first, while you are fresh. The next three stations can be ordered differently, however we recommend the Kettle-Bell Swings in the middle so that rotational and linear movements are alternated.

- The last two events are relatively safe (if form fails, there is no added weight to increase the injury risk), so you can push fatigue to the desired level.

Hines' Hell
30 seconds Bag Push
30 Seconds Isometric Squat Hold
30 Seconds Burpees
30 Seconds Rest

30 seconds Renegade Rows
30 seconds Push-ups on kettle bells
30 seconds mountain climbers on kettle bells
30 Seconds Rest

30 seconds Pull-Ups
30 seconds Isometric Holds at the Top of the Pull-Up bar.
30 seconds hanging leg raises
30 Seconds Rest

30 Seconds Kettle bell Cleans
30 Seconds Kettle bell Push-Presses
30 Seconds Air Squats
30 Seconds Rest

Then immediately start over at Bag Push.

Purpose: This workout does not fit neatly into one category. There is both a strong muscular endurance and anaerobic component.

Utilization: This is a stand-alone workout that is best suited as a Friday "Gut Check" for your men. Probably best to do this no more than once a month. The key is to go hard as you can and try not to pace yourself.

Precautions: When doing the Renegade Rows, be sure to keep the kettle bell directly under your armpit and lock-in before trying to row with the opposite arm. If you do not do this you risk the kettle bell rolling on your support arm and injuring your wrist.

Notes:
- Bag push refers to the Wave, water-filled device. You can substitute with sled push, Skedco drag, etc.
- Select a kettle bell weight you can Renegade Row for reps - usually 35-40 pounds. This will also be the weight you use for kettle bell cleans and push press.
- Three rounds is a hard workout. You can do four rounds if you really want to suffer. Do not do more than four rounds or you will lose intensity or sanity.
- To increase difficulty, simply go harder in each event and do more reps.

RNUT SPECIAL

The entire group completes 15 air squats, 10 push-ups, and 5 pull-ups as quickly as possible in a 1 minute timeframe. This usually takes 30-40 seconds. The remainder of the 1 minute will be rest and movement to the next station.

Then each Ranger will go to one of 4 stations

1) Tire Flips for 20m
2) Lateral jumps over orange cone or log
3) Med Ball Slams-20lb ball
4) Burpees

Persons at station 2, 3, 4 go as long as it takes the person doing tire flips to flip tire 20m.

Then repeat the 15 air squats, 10 push-up, and 5 pull-ups. Then rotate to the next station of the 4 stations listed about.

Continue for 10 rounds. You can do 15 rounds if you want to really push it.

Purpose: This workout is a nice hybrid work. There are components of strength endurance, agility and anaerobic fitness. One can adjust the volume and/or intensity to increase or decrease the difficulty of event. It is important to give maximum effort during each event. Pacing yourself can limit intent of the workout.

Utilization: This work out could be a stand-along workout, lasting about 30-45 minutes depending on the number of sets conducted. Consider doing it once a week for 3-4 weeks, increasing the volume along the way.

Precautions: The movements that make up this hybrid are pretty basic. Perform movement prep before this workout.

Notes:

- To increase difficulty, add additional reps or increase length of tire flip (there for increasing the length of each station).
- If there are a lot of Rangers, you can add more exercise stations.

Tactical PT

Effective physical training optimizes the ability to meet tactical physical requirements. In nearly all instances, these requirements demand a mix of movement skills, strength, and endurance. Rangers should establish good movement skills and a moderate to high level of strength and endurance before attempting O-courses and other very demanding tactical PT activities. Tactical PT events should be introduced during the Foundation Phase. Have a systematic plan for increasing the training stress (volume or intensity) over time.

Some recommended activities are:

- Traditional Obstacle Courses (various lengths and configurations): First, master standard obstacles in ACUs/Boots, then add RBA/MICH if it adds value and does not overly increase fall/injury risk.
- Combatives
- Casualty Evacuation Carries/Pulls
- Power Ruck: See Endurance section for details.
- Combination of the above. For example, lay out a course over several miles of varied terrain. Load and distance depend on progression within the training cycle. Place stations 1-2 km apart and include tire flips, litter carries, skedco pulls, sprints, etc.

Avoid overemphasis on any one mode of tactical training. Instead plan out your phased training schedule, to include all events at the appropriate time in the training cycle. *The first session of each tactical drill should be primarily instructional in nature.*

RAW Assessments

Introduction

Ranger missions require a broad range of physical attributes that can be grouped into three categories: Strength, Endurance, and Movement Skills. Within each category, the requirement is further defined as follows:

- Strength sufficient for load carriage, IMT, and CASEVAC without physical bulk that detracts from endurance or movement proficiency.
- Endurance sufficient for 1) long-range movement at a relatively low speed and 2) short, explosive movements followed by short rest and then repetition.
- Movement skills sufficient for the safe and effective execution of tasks that require power, agility, balance, and coordination

The primary purpose of the RAW assessments is to identify individual and team/squad areas needing improvement. This in turn guides subsequent physical training. The first seven tasks are athletic assessments that should be conducted twice during a complete training/deployment cycle; first during OP-PREP, then again during OP-ALERT. Tasks 1-7 **MUST** be conducted in order during a single, 90-minute PT session. Movement Prep as outlined in the RAW PT Manual, v4.0 is conducted immediately before the assessments. The RPAT is the primary tactical assessment, conducted once per training/deployment cycle and separate from any athletic assessment by at least two days.

In addition to following the task/conditions/standards below, leaders should document the weight of the Ranger and the conditions under which the assessments were conducted (temperature, humidity, wind, and condition of the field). Documenting the individual and team/squad scores can be facilitated by using the sample scorecards in Appendices A and B of this document. Note that the Functional Movement Screen (FMS) and BodPod (body composition expressed in percentage of body fat) scores can be documented on the individual scorecard. Those two tests are screening assessments and are conducted separate from the physical assessments listed below. The BN medical section coordinates the screening assessments.

TASK/CONDITIONS/STANDARDS

TASK 1: **5-10-5 Shuttle Run.** The purpose of this test is to measure quickness and agility.
CONDITIONS: Given a flat, athletic surface, with a length of 10 yards and three cones 5 yards apart from center.
STANDARDS: The Ranger straddles the middle cone. When the Ranger is ready, he will go into a three-point stance and start by going to the right and run five yards and touch the line with his right hand. He then turn and run 10 yards to his left and touch the other cone with his left hand. Ranger will then turn and run 5 yards through the center cone. The time is measured from when the Ranger makes his first movement to when he passes the start/stop line (the center cone). The test is repeated a second time going to the left. The better of the two times is the time that is recorded.

*Time is measured to the nearest tenth of a second (example: 5.6 seconds)

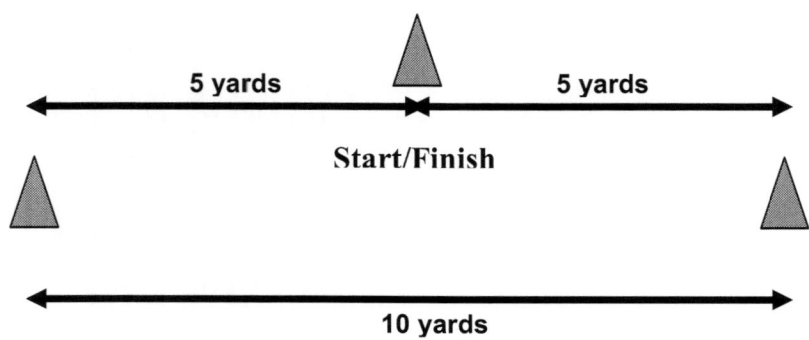

TASK 2: **Standing Broad Jump.** The purpose of this test is to measure total-body power.
CONDITIONS: Given a solid athletic surface, a tape measure, and a line to mark foot placement. Ranger will have two attempts to jump as far as they can. The better of the two attempts is recorded.
STANDARDS: Stand with toes behind the line. On each attempt, up to three preparatory movements are allowed. By the third prepatory movement, the Ranger will triple extend the knees, hips, and ankles while using the upper body to propel their body as far forward as possible. The Ranger must stick the landing. The measurement will be taken from the heel of the closest foot. The grader will record the farthest jump.

*Measure in Feet to nearest inch (example: 7ft 8in)

TASK 3: **225-pound Dead Lift.** The purpose of this test is to measure total-body lift strength from the ground.
CONDITIONS: Given a 45-lb Trap bar with two 45-lb plates loaded on each side for a total of 225 pounds.
STANDARDS: Stand inside the trap bar and lift the bar until standing erect. Foot and hand placement is of the Ranger's preference. Ensure grip is firm and is centered on the bar to prevent trap bar from going forward or backwards. At the top of the lift, the body must be perpendicular to the ground, without bend in the hips or knees. The grader states the number of the repetition at this point. If Ranger lowers the weight before achieving the fully erect stance, that repetition does not count. A pause in the up position of one second is allowed. Ranger will then lower the weight to the ground in a controlled manner. A slight pause is allowed while the weight is on the ground. Complete as many repetitions up to 30 repetitions. The event is terminated when Ranger reaches 30 repetition or if Ranger fails to maintain the proper cadence at the top or bottom of the lifts, drops the weight, or fails to maintain upward movement once a lift is started (i.e. hits a sticking point in the middle of a lift). The score is the number of correct repetitions performed. If a Ranger has never performed a dead lift, he should receive a zero or "N/A" for the event and be directed to meet with the BN HPOC to learn the proper mechanics of the dead lift.

TASK 4: Pull-up. The purpose of this test is to measure muscular strength and endurance of grip and upper body pulling muscles in relation to body weight.
CONDITIONS: Given a pull-up bar that allows full body extension without the feet touching the ground.
STANDARDS: On the command "Ready", move to a free-hang position with arms straight and elbows locked, using an overhand grip, with the thumbs placed over the bar. On the command of "GO", pull the body upward until the chin is over the bar. Return to the straight-arm hang position with his elbows locked. Repeat this pull-up movement as many times as possible. The body must maintain a generally straight plane from head to toe. If Ranger generates any type of momentum to complete the pull-up, the pull-up involved will not be counted. The grader may slow the speed of movement to ensure the elbows extend fully upon lowering. The score will be the number of correct repetitions performed.

TASK 5: Metronome Push-up. The purpose of this test is to measure the muscular endurance of upper body pushing and core muscles.
CONDITIONS: Given a solid, athletic surface and a metronome set to 1 second intervals.
STANDARDS: On the command "Get Ready," assume the kneeling front-leaning rest position. On the command "Get Set," assume the front-leaning rest position. On the command "GO," lower the body until the upper arm is parallel to the ground. On the next metronome sound, immediately return to the front-leaning rest. On the next metronome sound, immediately return to the lower position as described above. When Ranger can no longer stay with the metronome cadence, the test is terminated and the last number of correct reps is recorded. There are no rest positions for this test. The regular APFT standards are used to grade the push-up (i.e. body position, lower and upper position). The body must be maintained in a straight line throughout. If Ranger maintains the metronome cadence, but fails to meet other performance standards (i.e. does not extend elbows fully on rising, fails to bring the upper arms parallel to the ground on lowering, sags/arches the pelvis/trunk at any point) the grader will repeat the number of the last correct repetition and tell Ranger to make the proper correction. Alternately, the grader may give a tap on the arms or back to indicate the need go lower or keep the trunk straight.

TASK 6: Heel Clap. The purpose of this test is to measure muscular strength and endurance of grip, pulling, and core muscles.
CONDITIONS: Given a pull-up bar that allows full body extension without the feet touching the ground, and is long enough to allow the movement to standard.
STANDARDS: On the command, "Ready," Ranger moves to a free-hang position with elbows bent to approximately 90 degrees, using an alternating grip so that the body faces along the length of the pull-up bar rather than toward the bar. On the command "GO", Ranger lifts his lower body upward and raises the feet over the bar to tap the heels together (repetitions will not be counted if only the toes touch over the bar). He returns to the starting position, maintaining the elbows at 90 degrees throughout. He repeats this sequence as many times as possible. The body must be held approximately straight in the lower position. Ranger cannot rest the legs on the bar or swing past the starting position on lowering. If Ranger extends the elbows to less than 90 degrees, that repetition does not count. Ranger must return to and pause at 90 degrees before attempting the next repetition. Ranger's score will be the number of correct repetitions performed.

TASK 7: 300-yard Shuttle Run. The purpose of this test is to measure anaerobic endurance.
CONDITIONS: Given a flat, athletic surface with line markings 25 yards apart.
STANDARDS: Line up in the sprint, crouch, or standup start positions with both feet and hands behind the starting line. The grader will give a preparatory command, "Ready." On the command "GO", run to the opposite end of the course and make a direct turn by placing at least one foot on or over the line, return to the starting line, makes another turn, and continue in this way for **six round trips**, sprinting past the finish line on the last trip. Do not take a circular path to make any turn. The grader records the total time taken from their

command "Go" to completion of the course. A one-minute rest period is given, then the 300-yard shuttle is repeated. The rest period begins after the last Ranger in a group crosses the finish line. Leaders should organize the men so that there is minimal time separating the first and last Rangers in a group. The grader averages the two repetitions to calculate the overall score for this event.

*All times measured to nearest full second (ex: 62.4 sec = 62 sec and 62.5 = 63 sec)

TASK 8: **Ranger Physical Assessment Test (RPAT).** The purpose of this test is to measure all components of fitness (strength, endurance, movement skills), using tactically relevant tasks.
CONDITIONS: Given RBA, MICH helmet, and an obstacle course with a minimum of a 1 mile marked track, a 185lb Skedco, 20-foot fast rope apparatus, 20-foot caving ladder apparatus, and an 8-foot wall.
STANDARDS: Complete a 3-mile run and combat focused PT course in less than 1 hour. The event will be conducted at squad level, with the mindset that the Ranger is competing against himself. Each time the event is conducted, each Ranger should see constant improvement in his time and ability to negotiate the course.

2. Conduct a 2-mile run wearing ACUs, boots, RBA and MICH helmet.
3. After the completion of the run, climb the 20-foot fast rope and do a controlled descent.
3. Drag a 185-pound SKEDCO litter 50 yards, turn round and drag it back 50 yards to the start point.
4. Next, climb a 20-foot caving ladder and climb back down.
5. Then sprint 100 yards, turn around, sprint back 100 yards.
6. Scale an 8-foot wall.
7. Conduct a 1 mile run wearing ACUs, boots, RBA and MICH helmet. Time stops when you cross the line.

Training for the RAW Assessments

RAW assessments support the program's philosophy in several ways:

- Recognizing those Rangers with the best blend of strength, endurance, and movement skills
- Identifying individual areas of strength/weakness relative to other Rangers
- Guiding training decisions based on performance
- Promoting competition

To a large degree, simply following the training guidance provided in the RAW PT Manual, v3.0 will prepare Rangers for the assessments. The following information is meant to supplement that guidance and offer more specific suggestions for training. For information on how best to integrate these training suggestions into your overall workout plan, see the RAW SME-trained Rangers in the battalion or consult the Regimental RAW team.

1. 5-10-5 Pro Agility Test

Training: This test begins from the prone position, so the ability to move quickly out of the prone matters. Mountain climber sprints and plyometric pushups should help. While some agility tests have significant amounts of lateral movement, the Illinois test is more about stopping and starting. You have to be able to maintain sprint speed as far up to the turn points as possible. This means you need braking power and then acceleration. In training, explosive lunges will help with both the breaking and acceleration out of the flexed knee position. When performed on a regular basis, the power drill described in the RAW PT Manual should also help.

Technique: As for the actual technique of cutting around the cones in this assessment, the key is to use appropriate body lean to keep the center of the body inside the base of support (the feet, especially the outermost foot). For both safety and performance, get low when cutting.

2. Standing Broad Jump

Training: This is a test of total-body power. Power is a product of strength and speed. Because this assessment uses a relatively light weight, the speed component is very important. Plyometrics, hang cleans with a relatively light weight, and exercises from the RAW power drill should help. Of the many plyometric exercises, one that should have particular value for this assessment is the depth jump (step off of a platform, absorbing the impact with plenty of bend in the hips and knees, then with absolutely no pause at the bottom, jump straight up as high as possible...perform just a few reps with adequate rest between reps...perform after movement prep and before any fatiguing exercise). Training with a slightly heavier medicine ball might help; however, the size of the ball should be very similar.

Technique: Use two or three preparatory "swings" to get the movement grooved, then on the actual throw, move as fast as possible into and out of the squat. Keep the elbows extended to exert maximum leverage. If body lean and follow through are optimal, you should fall onto your back.

3. Dead Lift

Training: The dead lift mainly tests the strength of the legs, core, and grip. Exercises that can aide your dead lifting ability are squats, back extensions, rack pulls, and ground base dead lifts. Train without the use of lifting straps to develop adequate grip strength. There are two workouts that should be performed weekly. First, to stimulate the fast-twitch motor units involved with the dead lift, perform several sets with a weight that allows no more than four good reps. Rest between sets should be at least a couple minutes. Rest should be sufficient so that the weight need not be lowered during the later sets due to fatigue. The second workout should occur 3-4 days later and involve a weight that can be lifted 8-12 times. The rest between sets should be shorter so that the later sets are performed with some degree of fatigue. The weight for the later sets may be decreased in order to stay in the 8-12 rep range. For both of these workouts, perform at least a couple warm-up sets with a lighter weight, then perform 4-6 sets with the training weight.

Technique: Squat down and grasp the bar with an alternating grip slightly wider than shoulder width. Keeping your head up and back flat, drive your feet into the floor while contracting your abs and keep your core tight. Foot pressure should be greatest through the heel, not the toes. The bar should remain close to your body as you lift it. A repetition is complete when you stand completely erect. Lower the weight in a controlled manner until it touches floor. Do not let your back round or your weight shift forward to the balls of the feet because this could increase your chance of injury. Incorporate breathing by holding a full breath until you have passed through the most difficult part of the lift. Other methods, such as the sumo dead lift are also acceptable.

4. Pull-ups

Training: The pull-ups rely heavily on the lats and biceps. Exercises training those muscles, particularly in a combined pulling motion, will contribute to pulling strength. Lat pulls, dumbbell rows, and assisted pull ups (gravitron, elastic bands, or partner) are all good training options. If using assistance on the pull, go without assistance during the lowering phase. If you can already do 15 or more pull-ups, adding resistance with body armor or weights hanging from a lifting belt will help ensure you continue to develop more pulling strength.
Technique: Typically the best grip is shoulder-width or slightly wider. Ensure you use a thumbless grip when you train as this will be the same grip you use when you test. If you are doing weighted pull-ups, we recommend fully grasping the bar with your thumb to avoid slipping. Do not kip when preparing specifically for this assessment. Leaning back slightly can help engage other muscles in the back and allow you to squeeze out a few more reps.

5. Metronome Pushups

Training: The metronome style of pushup requires stabilizing effort of the core and shoulder girdle muscles throughout. There is no sagging/arching rest position, nor is there the brief unloaded moment that occurs with the momentum of fast-paced pushups. Therefore, core endurance exercises such as planks are helpful. Consistent with our philosophy of full-spectrum strength, training according to guidance in the strength section of the RAW PT Manual should help. Working heavy resistance, power-endurance, and body-weight endurance at least once every 7-10 days will ensure that all muscle fiber types that contribute to the metronome pushup are being trained.
Technique: Establish a tight core before the first repetition and maintain throughout. However, do not waste energy by squeezing the core so tight that breathing is altered. Incorporate the breathing cycle into repetitions – breathe in during the lowering and exhale on the way up. Do not waste energy going lower than is necessary.

6. Heel Claps

Training: This event requires isometric strength of the gripping and pulling muscles, as well as the trunk flexors. Consider training the isometric strength at the end of pull-up workouts. Improve trunk flexor strength for this task on an incline sit-up board, using the resistance of a plate/dumbbell/med ball/kettle bell at the chest or overhead. The weight used should permit no more than 20 good reps. Perform this exercise at a controlled speed because no momentum is allowed for the heel clap assessment.
Technique: The tilt of the pelvis may influence the potential strength of the trunk flexing muscles. From the hanging position, experiment with tilting the pelvis forward (belly and buttocks sticking out further than normal) or backward (belly and buttocks tucked in more than normal). Incorporate the breathing cycle into repetitions – breathe in during the lowering and exhale on the way up.

7. 300-Yard Shuttle Run

Training: This is primarily an anaerobic assessment, so just about any intense training where reps resume before recovery is complete will help. Sprints, intervals on the track, bike, rower, etc…Tabata intervals…hybrid workouts from X-Fit, Gym Jones…performing a couple of these each week will help. Because of the turns involved, training described for the Illinois Agility assessment should also help with shuttles runs.

Technique: Practice pacing to ensure more or less equal time for each segment. Practice turns to maximize efficiency. As with all cuts, lower your center of gravity and keep it inside the base of support. The work of braking your momentum and pushing off to change direction should be shared by both legs. Practice hop turns (180 degree change of body alignment occurs in the air) and pivot turns (place the plant foot parallel to the end line) to determine which method feels best for you. Do not round the turns.

Sample Assessment Scorecard

Ranger 1	FMS: 17/21	BodPod: 12% Body Fat
Performance Assessments	Raw Data Score	Squad Rank
5-10-5 Pro Agility	5.5 sec.	3
Standing Broad Jump	7ft 8 in	3
225lb Dead Lift	25 reps	4
Pull Up	15 reps	5
Metronome Push Up	48 reps	4
Heel Claps	18 reps	3
300yd Shuttle Run	69 sec	2
RPAT	34 min.	3
		AVG 3.4*

*Lowest score represents best overall fitness within the squad.

Sample Squad Data for a Single Event

300-Yard Shuttle Run (2 trials with 1-minute rest between)

	1st Trial (s)	2nd Trial (s)	Average	Squad Rank
Ranger 1	70	72	71	4
Ranger 2	71	74	72.5	6
Ranger 3	68	69	68.5	2
Ranger 4	74	77	75.5	10
Ranger 5	69	72	70.5	3
Ranger 6	70	72	71	4
Ranger 7	72	74	73	8
Ranger 8	73	75	74	9
Ranger 9	67	69	68	1
Ranger 10	71	74	72.5	6
Average	70.5	72.8	71.7*	

* Can be used for comparison between squads.

Sample Squad Overall Ranking	
	Squad Rank
Ranger 1	2.8
Ranger 2	3.2
Ranger 3	2.9
Ranger 4	7.2
Ranger 5	5.7
Ranger 6	4.4
Ranger 7	6.9
Ranger 8	6.9
Ranger 9	1.7*
Ranger 10	4.7

Olympic Lifts

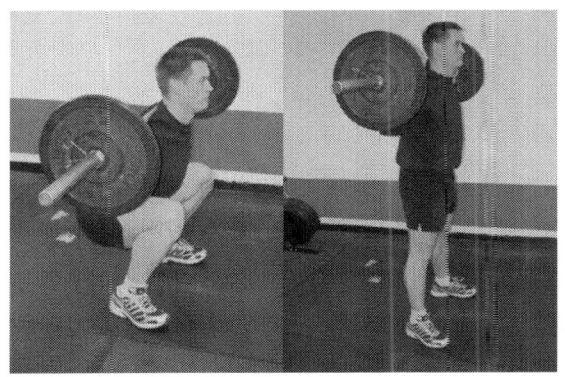

Back Squat:

Start Position—Grasp barbell from rack (barbell at upper chest height). Position barbell on back of shoulders and grasp bar to sides. Dismount bar from rack.

Execution—Lower body until hips and knees are fully bent or until thighs are just past parallel to floor. Ensure knees stay over the feet by thrusting buttocks to the rear as if sitting in a chair. Allow hips to bend back behind knees. Keep back straight and knees pointed same direction as feet. Then extend knees and hips simultaneously until legs are straight.

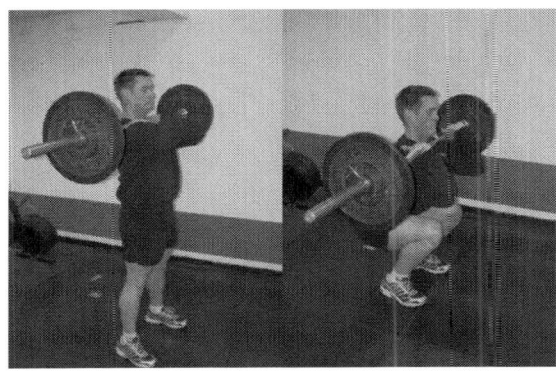

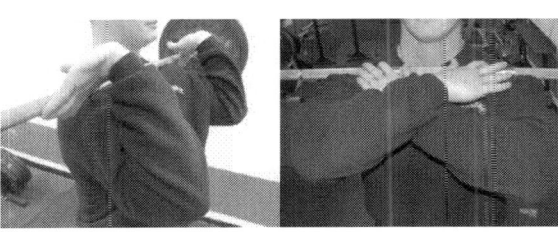

Front Squat:

Start Position—Grasp barbell from rack or clean barbell from floor with overhand open grip. Grip should be slightly wider than shoulder width. Place bar in front of shoulders with elbows placed forward as high as possible and finger under bar to each side. Alternate grip with hands touching opposite shoulder can also be used. With heels hip width or slightly wider, position feet outward at approximately 45°.

Execution—Lower body until knees and hips are fully bent or until thighs are just past parallel to floor. Ensure knees stay over the feet by thrusting buttocks to the rear as if sitting in a chair. Allow hips to bend back behind knees. Keep back straight and knees pointed same direction as feet. Then extend knees and hips simultaneously until legs are straight.

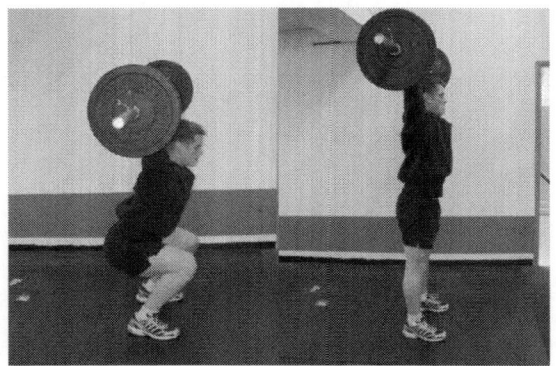

Overhead Squat:

Start Position—clean or Press barbell overhead with wide overhand grip. Position toes outward with wide stance. Maintain bar behind head with arms extended.

Execution— Lower body until knees and hips are fully bent or until thighs are just past parallel to floor. Ensure knees stay over the feet by thrusting buttocks to the rear as if sitting in a chair. Allow hips to bend back behind knees. Keep back straight and knees pointed same direction as feet. Ensure arms are fully extended with bar behind the head. Then extend knees and hips simultaneously until legs are straight.

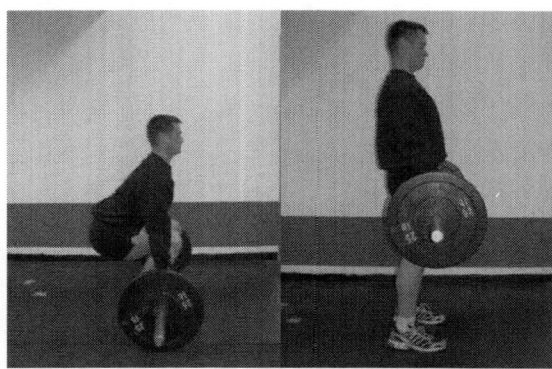

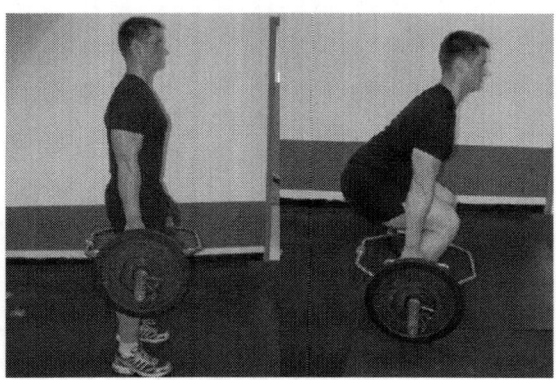

Dead Lift:

Start Position—Ensure feet are under the bar, the back straight, shoulders pulled back and aligned over the bar, heels down, hips low, head and chest up, and arms outside the legs. The reverse grip is recommended for heavier weights.

Execution—Raise the bar by pushing through the heels to rise to a fully upright stance. Keep the bar as close to the body as possible. Attempt to rise as a unit, rather than with the hips first, then the upper body. There is no need to lean backward at the top.

Optional Trap Bar Dead Lift

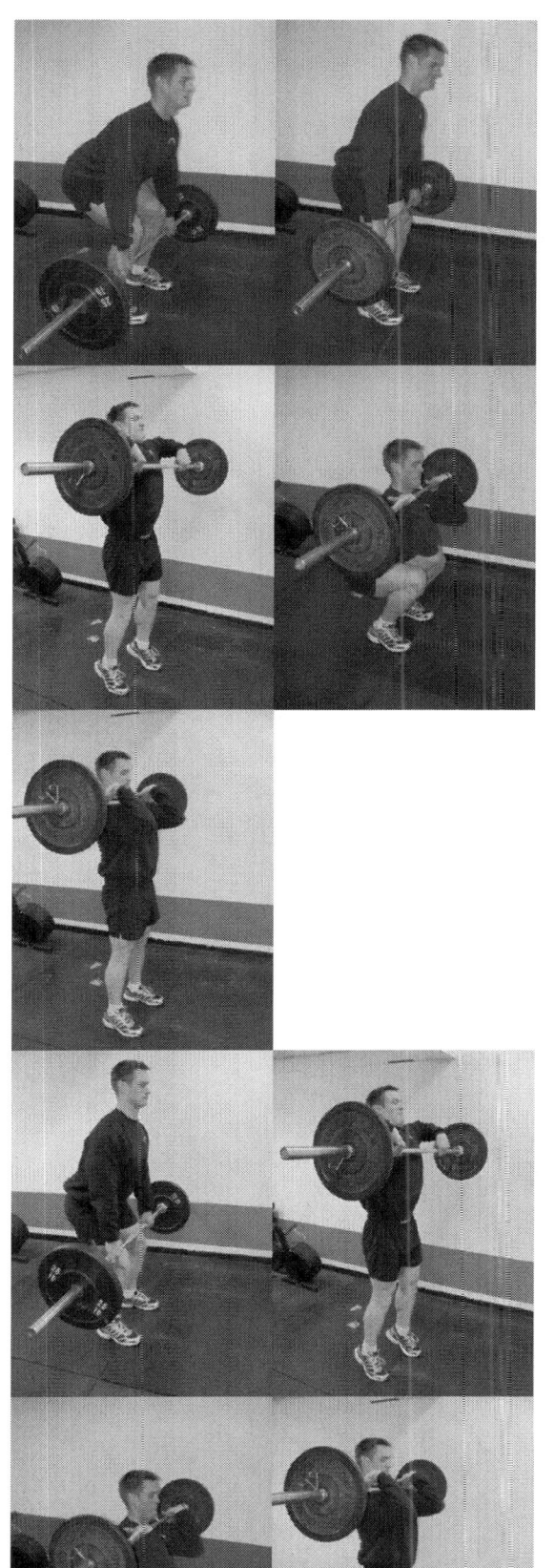

Power Clean:

Start Position—Stand over barbell with balls of feet positioned under bar pointing forward, hip width's apart or slightly wider. Squat down and grip bar with over hand grip slightly wider than shoulder width. Position shoulders over bar with back arched tightly. Arms are straight with elbows pointed along bar

Execution—Pull bar up off floor by extending hips and knees. As bar reaches knees vigorously raise shoulders while keeping barbell close to thighs. When barbell passes mid-thigh, allow it to contact thighs. Jump upward extending body (triple extension through the hips, knees, and ankles). Shrug shoulders and pull barbell upward with arms allowing elbows to flex out to sides, keeping bar close to body. Aggressively pull body under bar, rotating elbows around bar. Catch bar on shoulders while moving into squat position. Hitting bottom of squat, stand up immediately.

Return—Bend knees slightly and lower barbell to mid-thigh position. Slowly lower bar to the ground.

Hang Clean:

Start Position—Stand with barbell using and overhand grip slightly wider than shoulder width. Feet should point forward, hip's width apart or slightly wider. Bend knees and hips so barbell touches just above the knee; shoulders over bar. Arms are straight with elbows pointed along bar.

Execution— Back tight at all times. Hold bar slightly less than thumb distance from knurling. Elbows rotated out to keep your arms straight at all times. This is a leg movement, not an arm movement; keep your arms straight at all times. Bend the knees 2-3" keeping the shoulders and back vertical and pause. Bend forward by pushing the butt out and back in order to get your shoulders n front of the bar. Jump and shrug while keeping your arms straight. This jump and shrug gets the bar moving upward. Once your jump is completed and the bar is accelerating upward you catch the bar by stomping your feet on the ground while driving the elbows down and thru to catch the bar at shoulder level.
Return—Bend knees slightly and lower barbell to mid-thigh position.

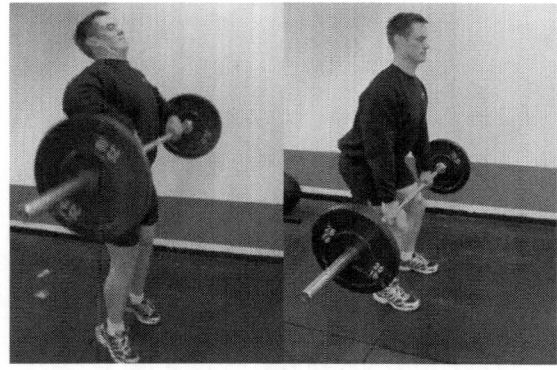

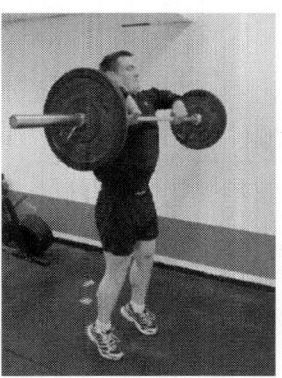

High Pull:

Start Position—Stand over barbell with balls of feet positioned under bar slightly wider apart than hip width. Squat down and grip bar with over hand grip slightly wider than shoulder width. Position shoulders over bar with back arched tightly. Arms are straight with elbows pointed along bar.

Execution-- Pull bar up off floor by extending hips and knees. As bar reaches knees vigorously raise shoulders while keeping barbell close to thighs, jump upward extending body. Flex elbows out to sides, pulling bar up to neck height.

Return—Bend knees slightly and lower barbell to mid-thigh position. Slowly lower bar with taut lower back and trunk close to vertical. The advanced athlete may *unload* (drop) bar from completed position. This technique may be practiced to reduce stress or fatigue involved in lowering bar as prescribed.

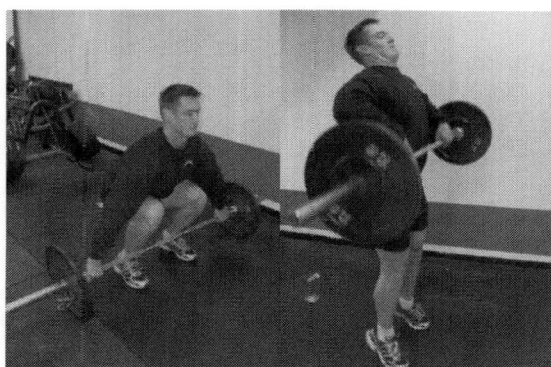

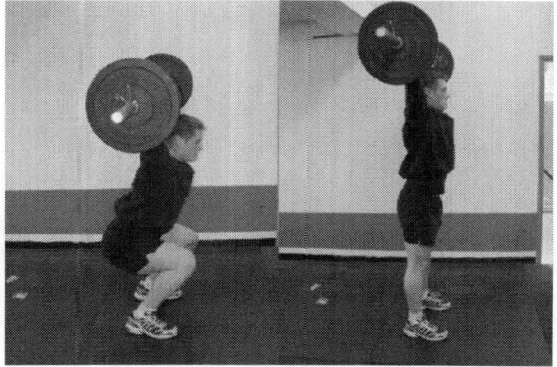

Snatch:

Start Position—Stand over barbell with balls of feet positioned under bar hip width or slightly wider than hip width apart. Squat down and grip bar with very wide over hand grip. Position shoulders over bar with back arched tightly. Arms are straight with elbows pointed along bar.

Execution—Pull bar up off floor by extending hips and knees. As bar reaches knees back stays arched and maintains same angle to floor as in starting position. When barbell passes knees, explode raise shoulders while keeping bar as close to legs as possible. When bar passes upper thighs allow it to contact thighs. Explode upward extending body. Shrug shoulders and pull barbell upward with arms allowing elbows to pull up to sides, keeping them over bar as long as possible. Aggressively pull body under bar. Catch bar at arm's length while moving into squat position. As soon as barbell is caught on locked arms in squat position, squat up into standing position with barbell overhead.

Return—Bend knees slightly and lower barbell to mid-thigh position. Slowly lower bar with taut lower back and trunk close to vertical. The advanced athlete may *unload* (drop) bar from completed position. This technique may be practiced to reduce stress or fatigue involved in lowering bar as prescribed.

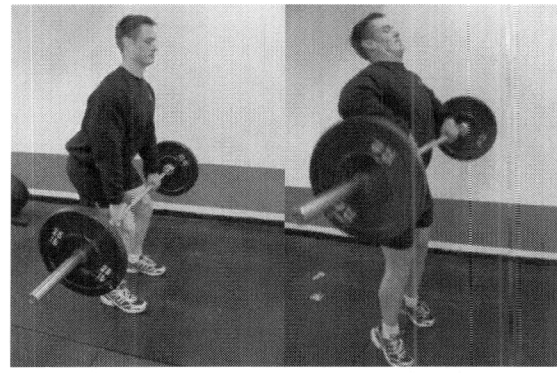

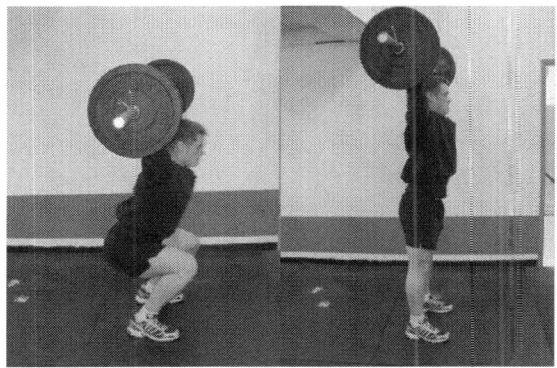

Hang Snatch:

Start Position—Stand with barbell with very wide over hand grip. Bend knees and hips so barbell touches upper-thigh; shoulders over bar with back arched. Arms are straight with elbows pointed along bar.

Execution—Jump upward extending body. Shrug shoulders and pull barbell upward with arms allowing elbows to pull up to sides, keeping them over bar as long as possible Aggressively pull body under bar. Catch bar at arm's length while moving into squat position. As soon as barbell is caught on locked out arms in squat position, squat up into standing position with barbell overhead.

Return—Bend knees slightly and lower barbell to mid-thigh position.

Kettebell Exercises

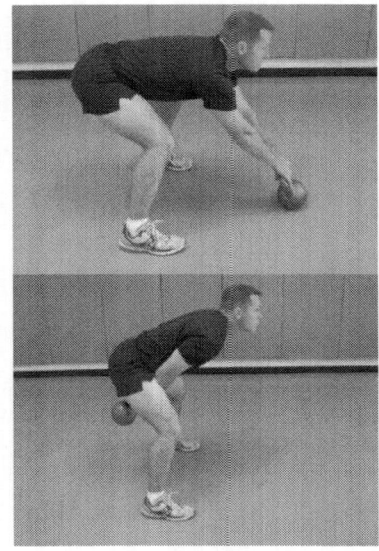

Two-Arm Kettlebell Swing:

Start Position—Stand one foot behind kettlebell, grasping KB with both hands, loading the hamstrings with a good athletic posture.

Execution—Throw KB in a 'hiking' motion between the legs maintaining a good athletic posture. This loads the body. Then triple extend the hips, knees, and ankles in an explosive manner. At this time, the arms should serve as a tether, only guiding the KB to about eye level. The height of the KB is dictated by the explosiveness of the lower body.

Return—Lower the KB by using gravity to control the KB back into the athletic position with the KB high in the crotch (ie. a witch on a broomstick).

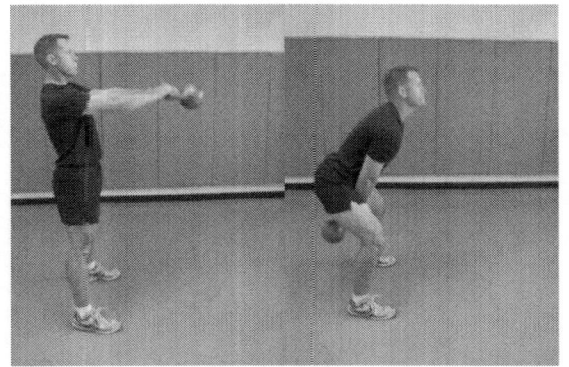

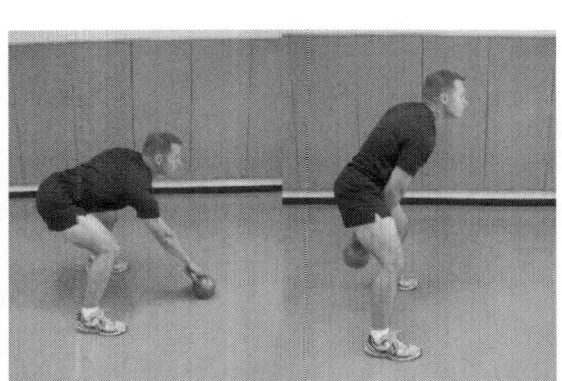

One-Arm KB Swing:

Start Position: Same position as the Two-Arm KB Swing except the free arm is to the side.

Execution—Same as Two-Arm swing. Ensure to "pop" the hips. Do NOT support body by placing free hand on thigh.

Return—Same as Two-Arm KB Swing

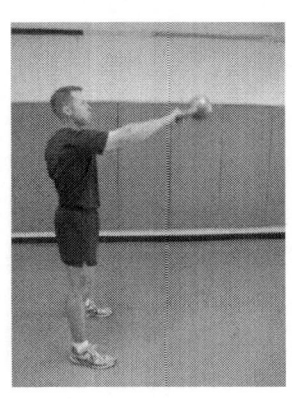

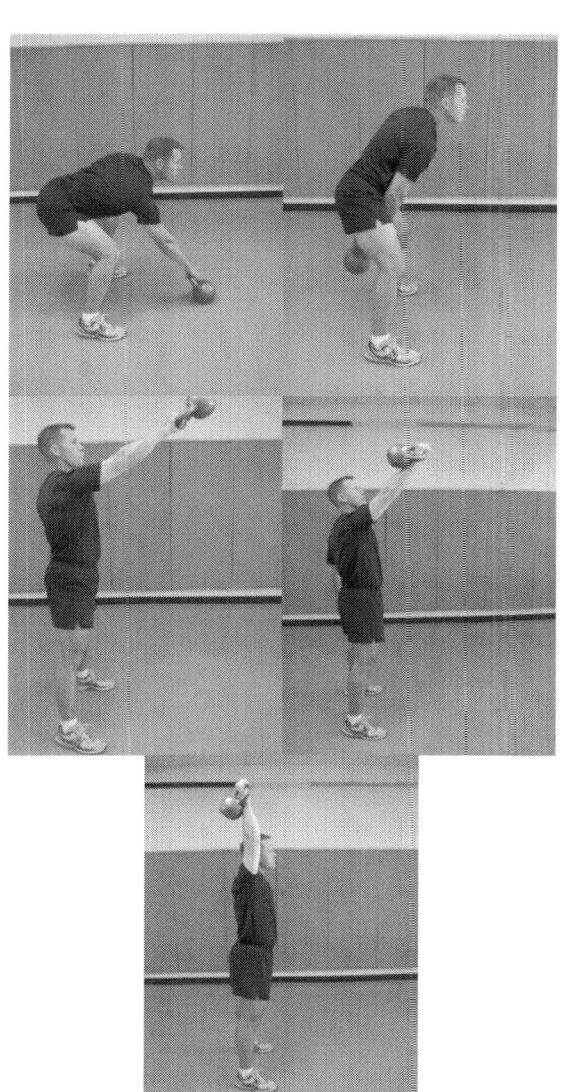

Kettlebell Snatch:

Start Position— Stand one foot behind kettlebell, grasping KB with one hand, loading the hamstrings with a good athletic posture.

Execution—Throw KB in a 'hiking' motion between the legs maintaining a good athletic posture. This loads the body. Then triple extend the hips, knees, and ankles in an explosive manner. At this time, the arm should serve as a tether, only guiding the KB to about eye level. This is when the front of the arm is engaged to continue raising the KB. Approximately at head level, slightly retract the shoulder and slightly flex the elbow and the punch the arm toward the sky while simultaneously moving the arm to the fully extended position by the ear. This movement will prevent the KB from banging on the forearm.

Return—Lower the KB by using gravity to control the KB back into the athletic position with the KB high in the crotch (ie. a witch on a broomstick). This will load the body in preparation for the next repetition

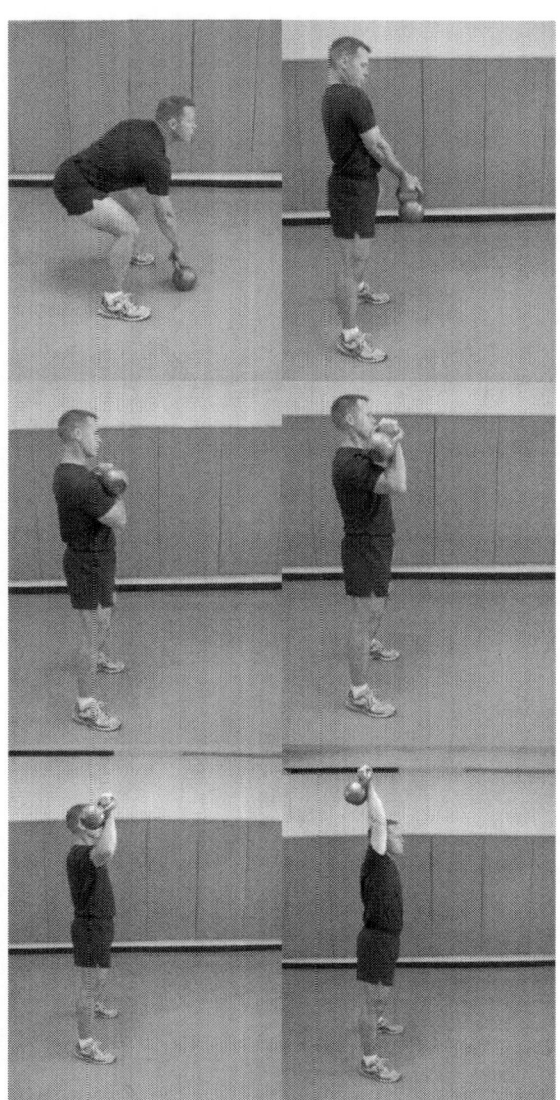

Kettlebell Clean and Press

Start Position—Begin with KB one foot in front. Maintain good athletic position.

Execution—Hike KB slightly between leg and extend hips and knees. Maintain KB close to body. Upward movement of hand should be similar to an "uppercut." Punch should end with elbow tight to side, KB in rack position, and fist in the center of chest under chin. Wrist should remain straight throughout the movement. Do NOT allow wrist to hyperextend. Next, open the shoulder and press KB upwards until elbow and shoulder are fully extended. End position is arm fully extended with arm next to the ear.

Return—Lower KB down to rack position. Ensure elbow is tight to side, wrist straight, and KB in nook of elbow.

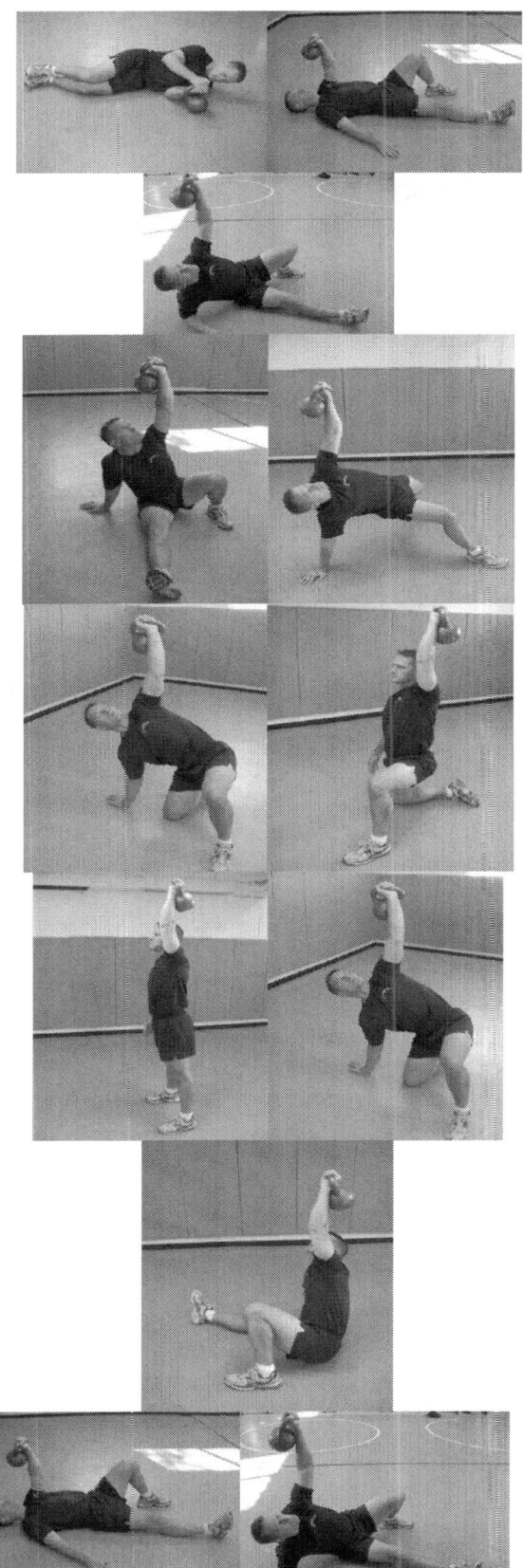

Kettlebell Turkish Get-Up:

Start Position—While on side, grasp KB with both hands and roll to back. Press KB until elbow is straight. Ensure wrist stays straight during entire movement. Bend the knee on the same side as the KB. Opposite arm is at a 45 degree angle from the body. Keep eyes on KB during entire movement unless directed otherwise.

Execution—Punch and crunch in the direction of the 45 degree arm until supported on elbow. Then extend elbow to supported position on hand. Do NOT move hand or arm during this movement. Once on hand, extend hips into a high bridge position. Sweep opposite leg to the midpoint of hand and leg. Shoulders should be stacked in a supported position. Flex side until trunk is in an upright posture and on one knee. At this time eyes can focus on the horizon and then go to a standing position. Lower body to the same one knee position as earlier. At this time, eyes need to be focused on KB. Place palm 6-8 inches to the outside of knee. Should be in the same stacked position as earlier. Extend downed knee to front. Two options here: 1) Go to high bridge and then lower to buttocks. 2) Go directly to buttocks. Lower body to elbow position. Then lower to supine position.

Keys:
    -Movement should be slow and deliberate. Move at a Tai-Chi pace or take a 1 second pause after each movement.
    -Elbow needs to be in a fully locked position at all times to ensure shoulder stabilizers are being targeted.
    -Do not move arm once placed at a 45 degree angle. This ensures movement to the arm and more effectively engages the core.

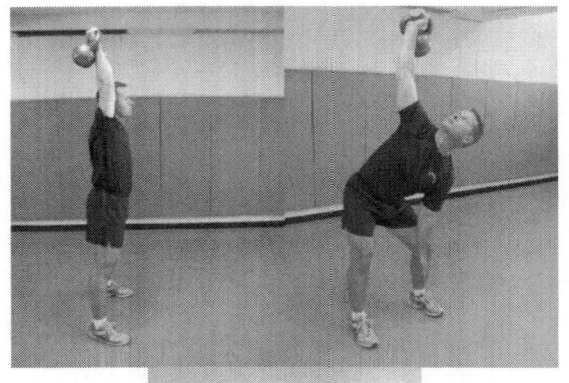

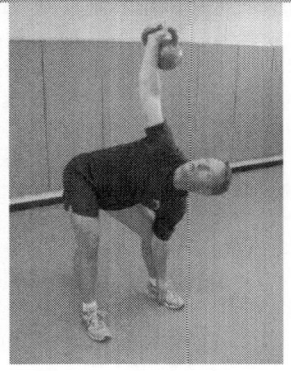

Kettlebell Windmill:

Start Position—Standing position with KB overhead, arm fully extended, wrist straight, and eyes looking straight ahead

Execution—With eyes on the KB, begin to rotate the core and drive the opposite arm down the inside of the leg towards the ground. The end position should be shoulders stacked on top of one another (similar to the Turkish Get-Up) with eyes focused on KB. Return to upright standing position.

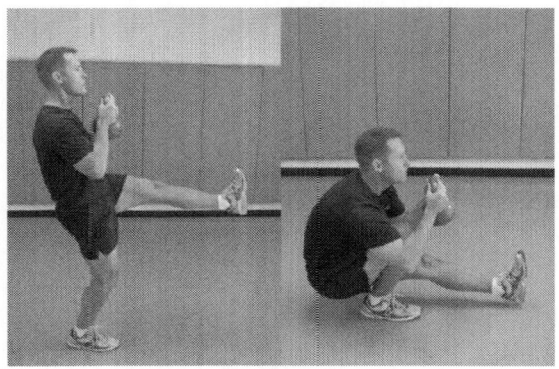

Kettlebell Pistol Squat:

Start Position—Begin in an upright with one leg extended forward. Flex hip fully and maintain full extension at knee. Maintain two handed grip on KB with KB close to chest.

Execution—Lower body into a deep squat position in a controlled manner. Pause in the down position and then

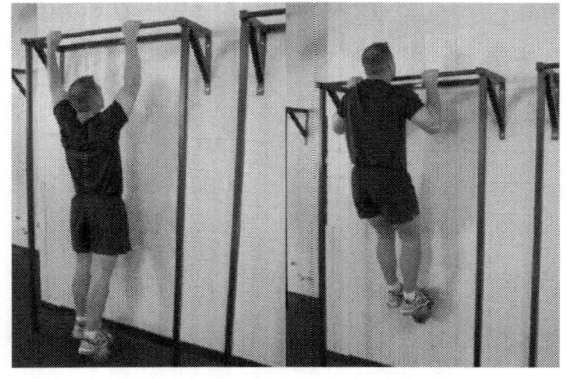

Kettlebell Pull-up:

Start Position—Begin in full hanging position with arms fully extended with foot inserted into KB handle. Toes/foot pointing toward sky (dorsiflexed) to maintain KB on foot. Multiple grips can be utilized depending upon intent of workout

Execution—Pull body upwards until chin is above bar. Do not kip. Lower body slowly back to starting position.

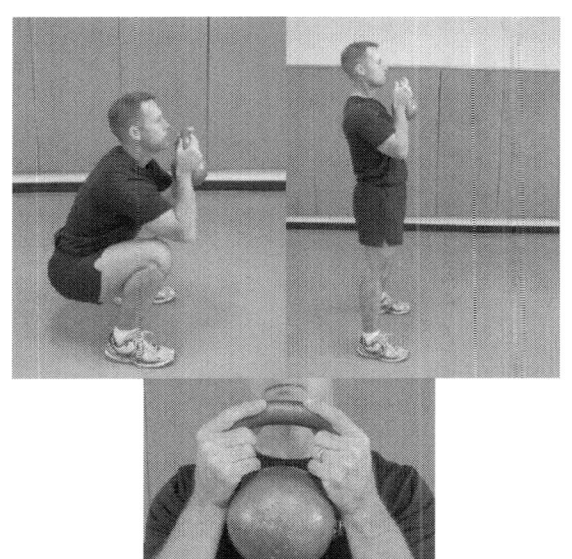

Kettlebell Goblet Squat:

Start Position—Grasp KB by handles using both hands. Feet shoulder width with feet pointing forward. Maintain KB close to chest.

Execution— Lower body until knees and hips are fully bent or until thighs are just past parallel to floor. Ensure knees stay over the feet by thrusting buttocks to the rear as if sitting in a chair. Allow hips to bend back behind knees. Keep back straight and knees pointed same direction as feet. Then extend knees and hips simultaneously until legs are straight.

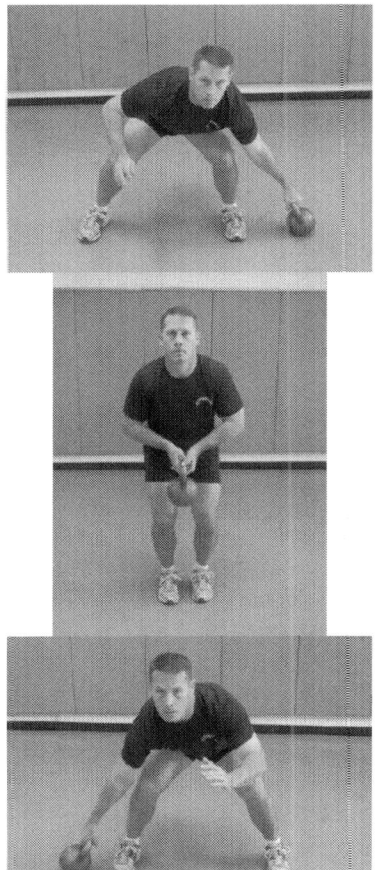

Kettlebell Lateral Drill:

Start Position—Get in a good athletic position. Place KB on the outside of foot, approximately 8 inches from foot. Opposite hand should be in front of body, not resting on thigh. Ensure knee on the side of the KB stays inside of the corresponding ankle.

Execution—Begin exercise by extending hips, knees, and ankles slightly into a ready position and shuttle laterally while transferring the KB from the outside position to the midline of body. Ensure to maintain a straight back, butt back, and head up. Transition KB to the opposite hand to the outside of opposite foot and touch KB to the ground. Repeat the opposite direction for a full repetition.

Transition Phase #1
Sample 3W Schedule

	MON	TUE	WED	THU	FRI
W1	1. 30 min Run 2. Core	Strength TNG: Endurance Emphasis	1. Speed & Agility 2. 30-30s	Alternative Cardio (swim, bike, row, etc)	Strength TNG: Power or Power-Endurance
W2	1. 30 min Run 2. Core	Strength TNG: Endurance Emphasis	1. Speed & Agility 2. 30-30s	Alternative Cardio (swim, bike, row, etc)	Strength TNG: Heavy Resistance
W3	RAW Assessments	Strength TNG: Endurance Emphasis	1. Speed & Agility 2. 30-30s	Alternative Cardio (swim, bike, row, etc)	Strength TNG: Power or Power-Endurance

•If only **four PT sessions** are available for a given week, alternate days that emphasize endurance with days that emphasize strength.

•If only **three PT sessions** are available for a given week, the preferred choice is two sessions that emphasize endurance and one strength.

•If only **two PT** sessions are available for a given week, perform one endurance workout and one strength workout.

Foundation Phase
Sample Schedule 1st Month

	MON	TUE	WED	THU	FRI
W1	1. 30 min Run 2. Core	Strength TNG: Heavy Resistance	1. Power Drill 2. 30-30s	Strength TNG: Power or Power-Endurance	Alternative Cardio (swim, bike, row, etc)
W2	1. 30 min Run 2. Core	Strength TNG: Heavy Resistance	1. Speed & Agility 2. 30-30s	Strength TNG: Endurance Emphasis	Footmarch or Tactical PT
W3	1. 35 min Run 2. Core	Strength TNG: Power or Power-Endurance	1. Power Drill 2. 30-30s	Strength TNG: Heavy Resistance	Alternative Cardio (swim, bike, row, etc)
W4	1. 35 min Run 2. Core	Strength TNG: Power or Power-Endurance	1. Speed & Agility 2. 30-30s	Strength TNG: Endurance Emphasis	Footmarch or Tactical PT

•If only **four PT sessions** are available for a given week, alternate days that emphasize endurance with days that emphasize strength.

•If only **three PT sessions** are available for a given week, the preferred choice is two sessions that emphasize endurance and one strength.

•If only **two PT** sessions are available for a given week, perform one endurance workout and one strength workout.

Foundation Phase
Sample Schedule 2nd Month

	MON	TUE	WED	THU	FRI
W1	1. 35 min Run 2. Core	Strength TNG: Heavy Resistance	1. Intervals 2. Core	Strength TNG: Power or Power-Endurance	Alternative Cardio (swim, bike, row, etc)
W2	1. 40 min Run 2. Core	Strength TNG: Heavy Resistance	1. Agility 2. Intervals	Strength TNG: Endurance Emphasis	Footmarch or Tactical PT
W3	1. 40 min Run 2. Core	Strength TNG: Power or Power-Endurance	1. Intervals 2. Core	Strength TNG: Heavy Resistance	Alternative Cardio (swim, bike, row, etc)
W4	1. 40 min Run 2. Core	Strength TNG: Power or Power-Endurance	1. Agility 2. Intervals	Strength TNG: Endurance Emphasis	Footmarch or Tactical PT

•If only **four PT sessions** are available for a given week, alternate days that emphasize endurance with days that emphasize strength.
•If only **three PT sessions** are available for a given week, the preferred choice is two sessions that emphasize endurance and one strength.
•If only **two PT** sessions are available for a given week, perform one endurance workout and one strength workout.

Foundation Phase
Sample Schedule 3rd Month

	MON	TUE	WED	THU	FRI
W1	1. 40+ min Run 2. Core	Strength TNG: Heavy Resistance	1. Intervals 2. Core	Strength TNG: Power or Power-Endurance	Alternative Cardio (swim, bike, row, etc)
W2	1. 40+ min Run 2. Core	Strength TNG: Heavy Resistance	1. Agility 2. Intervals	Strength TNG: Endurance Emphasis	Footmarch or Tactical PT
W3	1. 40+ min Run 2. Core	Strength TNG: Power or Power-Endurance	1. Intervals 2. Core	Strength TNG: Heavy Resistance	Alternative Cardio (swim, bike, row, etc)
W4	1. 40+ min Run 2. Core	Strength TNG: Power or Power-Endurance	1. Agility 2. Intervals	Strength TNG: Endurance Emphasis	Footmarch or Tactical PT

•If only **four PT sessions** are available for a given week, alternate days that emphasize endurance with days that emphasize strength.
•If only **three PT sessions** are available for a given week, the preferred choice is two sessions that emphasize endurance and one strength.
•If only **two PT** sessions are available for a given week, perform one endurance workout and one strength

Endurance Phase
Sample Schedule 1st Month

	MON	TUE	WED	THU	FRI
W1	1. 40+ min Run 2. Core	Strength TNG: Power-Endurance	1. Long Intervals 2. Core	Strength TNG: Endurance Emphasis	Terrain Run
W2	1. 40+ min Run 2. Core	Strength TNG: Heavy Resistance	1. Long Intervals 2. Core	Strength TNG: Endurance Emphasis	Footmarch or Tactical PT
W3	1. 40+ min Run 2. Core	Strength TNG: Power-Endurance	1. Agility 2. 20-min Tempo Run	Strength TNG: Endurance Emphasis	Alternative Cardio (swim, bike, row, etc)
W4	1. 40+ min Run 2. Core	Strength TNG: Power-Endurance	1. Long Intervals 2. Core	Strength TNG: Endurance Emphasis	Footmarch or Tactical PT

•If only **four PT sessions** are available for a given week, alternate days that emphasize endurance with days that emphasize strength.
•If only **three PT sessions** are available for a given week, the preferred choice is two sessions that emphasize endurance and one strength.
•If only **two PT** sessions are available for a given week, perform one endurance workout and one strength workout.

Endurance Phase
Sample Schedule 2nd Month

	MON	TUE	WED	THU	FRI
W1	1. 40+ min Run 2. Core	Strength TNG: Heavy Resistance	1. Long Intervals 2. Core	Strength TNG: Endurance Emphasis	Terrain Run
W2	1. 40+ min Run 2. Core	Strength TNG: Power-Endurance	1. Long Intervals 2. Core	Strength TNG: Endurance Emphasis	Footmarch or Tactical PT
W3	1. 40+ min Run 2. Core	Strength TNG: Power-Endurance	1. Agility 2. 20-min Tempo Run	Strength TNG: Endurance Emphasis	Alternative Cardio (swim, bike, row, etc)
W4	RAW Assessments	Strength TNG: Heavy Resistance	1. Long Intervals 2. Core	Strength TNG: Endurance Emphasis	Footmarch or Tactical PT

•If only **four PT sessions** are available for a given week, alternate days that emphasize endurance with days that emphasize strength.
•If only **three PT sessions** are available for a given week, the preferred choice is two sessions that emphasize endurance and one strength.
•If only **two PT** sessions are available for a given week, perform one endurance workout and one strength workout.

Transition Phase #2
Sample 3W Schedule

	MON	TUE	WED	THU	FRI
W1	1. 30 min Run 2. Core	Strength TNG: Power or Power-Endurance	1. Speed & Agility 2. 30-30s	Strength TNG: Endurance Emphasis	Terrain Run
W2	1. 30-60 min Run 2. Core	Strength TNG: Heavy Resistance	1. Speed & Agility 2. 300-yard Shuttle Repeats	Strength TNG: Power or Power-Endurance	Footmarch or Tactical PT
W3	1. 30 min Run 2. Core	Strength TNG: Endurance Emphasis	1. Agility 2. 20-min Tempo Run	Strength TNG: Power or Hybrid for Power-Endurance	Alternative Cardio (swim, bike, row, etc)

- If only **four PT sessions** are available for a given week, alternate days that emphasize endurance with days that emphasize strength.
- If only **three PT sessions** are available for a given week, the preferred choice is two sessions that emphasize endurance and one strength.
- If only **two PT** sessions are available for a given week, perform one endurance workout and one strength workout.

Strength Phase
Sample Schedule 1st Month

	MON	TUE	WED	THU	FRI	SAT	SUN
W1	Strength TNG: Mod-Heavy Resistance Legs/Back	Rest	1. Strength TNG: Mod-Heavy Upper Body 2. Cardio	Strength TNG: Power or Power-Endurance	Cardio Machines	Strength TNG: Mod-Heavy Resistance Total Body	Rest
W2	Strength TNG: Mod-Heavy Resistance Legs/Back	Rest	1. Strength TNG: Mod-Heavy Upper Body 2. Cardio	Strength TNG: Power or Power-Endurance	Cardio Machines	Strength TNG: Mod-Heavy Resistance Total Body	Rest
W3	Strength TNG: Mod-Heavy Resistance Legs/Back	Rest	1. Strength TNG: Mod-Heavy Upper Body 2. Cardio	Strength TNG: Power or Power-Endurance	Cardio Machines	Strength TNG: Mod-Heavy Resistance Total Body	Rest
W4	Strength TNG: Mod-Heavy Resistance Legs/Back	Rest	1. Strength TNG: Mod-Heavy Upper Body 2. Cardio	Strength TNG: Power or Power-Endurance	Cardio Machines	Strength TNG: Endurance Emphasis	Rest

Strength Phase
Sample Schedule 2nd Month

	MON	TUE	WED	THU	FRI	SAT	SUN
W 1	Strength TNG: Heavy Resistance Legs/Back	Rest	1. Strength TNG: Heavy Upper Body 2. Cardio	Strength TNG: Power or Power-Endurance	Cardio Machines	Strength TNG: Heavy Resistance Total Body	Rest
W 2	Strength TNG: Heavy Resistance Legs/Back	Rest	1. Strength TNG: Heavy Upper Body 2. Cardio	Strength TNG: Power or Power-Endurance	Cardio Machines	Strength TNG: Heavy Resistance Total Body	Rest
W 3	Strength TNG: Heavy Resistance Legs/Back	Rest	1. Strength TNG: Heavy Upper Body 2. Cardio	Strength TNG: Power or Power-Endurance	Cardio Machines	Strength TNG: Heavy Resistance Total Body	Rest
W 4	Strength TNG: Heavy Resistance Legs/Back	Rest	1. Strength TNG: Heavy Upper Body 2. Cardio	Strength TNG: Power or Power-Endurance	Cardio Machines	Strength TNG: Endurance Emphasis	Rest

Strength Phase
Sample Schedule 3rd Month

	MON	TUE	WED	THU	FRI	SAT	SUN
W 1	Strength TNG: Heavy Resistance Legs/Back	Rest	1. Strength TNG: Heavy Upper Body 2. Cardio	Strength TNG: Power or Power-Endurance	Cardio Machines	Strength TNG: Heavy Resistance Total Body	Rest
W 2	Strength TNG: Heavy Resistance Legs/Back	Rest	1. Strength TNG: Heavy Upper Body 2. Cardio	Strength TNG: Power or Power-Endurance	Cardio Machines	Strength TNG: Heavy Resistance Total Body	Rest
W 3	Strength TNG: Heavy Resistance Legs/Back	Rest	1. Strength TNG: Heavy Upper Body 2. Cardio	Strength TNG: Power or Power-Endurance	Cardio Machines	Strength TNG: Heavy Resistance Total Body	Rest
W 4	Strength TNG: Heavy Resistance Legs/Back	Rest	1. Strength TNG: Heavy Upper Body 2. Cardio	Strength TNG: Power or Power-Endurance	Cardio Machines	Strength TNG: Endurance Emphasis	Rest

OTHER OPTIONS

General Purpose, 6-Day Rotating Schedule					
PT1	PT2	PT3	PT4	PT5	PT6
Movement Preparation/Warm-Up (10 minutes)					
•Choose event from Strength Menu* **and/or** •Choose a Hybrid Session* **and/or** •Secondary Run **or** •Swimming	•Choose from Endurance Menu* **and** •Choose from Core Menu*	•Power-Endurance (Ground Base or Hybrid) **and** •Speed & Agility &/or Power Drill **and** •Partner Shuttle	•Interval Run (30/30s, intervals) **and** •Choose from Core Menu*	•Choose from Strength Menu* **or** •Choose from Hybrid or Tactical* **and/or** •Secondary Run **or** •Swimming	•Company-directed PT with endurance emphasis: -Hybrid -Tactical -Swim -Run -Cardio equipment -Footmarch
Recovery Activities/Cool-Down (10-12 minutes)					
*See RAW Events Chart and Menus on next slide					

Physical Training Events	
Movement Skills	
Movement Prep Speed/Agility/Coordination Power Drill Recovery Drill Flexibility	
--	
Core Strength Menu	
360-Core Med Ball Drills	
Endurance Menu	**Strength Menu**
Primary Runs • Steady-pace Run • Interval Run Ex: 30/30s, track intervals • Tempo Run • Fartlek Run **Secondary Runs** • 300-yd Shuttles • Terrain Run Foot march (variable parameters) Swimming or Deep-Water Running Bike or Cardio Machines	Heavy Resistance Power Power Endurance Muscular Endurance
Hybrid Sessions and Tactical PT	
See the RAW PT Manual for details.	

RAW 2-week Gym-based Workouts

- RAW Movement Prep prior to all workouts
- RAW Mobility/Flexibility drills after all workouts
- Recommended workout days: MON, TUES, WED, FRI, SAT
- Recommended rest days: THURS, SUN
    - Note: Rest = no workout at all

Workout 1

	Exercise	Sets	Reps	Rest
1	Deadlift	1+4	6	3min
2	One-arm Pull-ups	4	6	3min
3	Standing OH Bar Press	4	6	3min
4	Goblet Squat	4	6	3min
5	Weighted Pull-ups	4	6	3min
6	Weighted Dips	4	6	3min

Workout 2

- Take your 5 mile run time and convert it to seconds
- Divide that by 10 and then subtract 15 seconds
- The number you get with the second bullet is your target time (no faster, Ranger) for each 800 meter sprint that you'll run, 10 times, with 60 seconds of rest in between each sprint.

Workout 3

	Exercise	Sets	Reps	Rest
1	Front Squat	1+4	6	3min
2	One Arm Push-ups	4	6	3min
3	Weighted Chin-ups	4	6	3min
4	Single-leg DB Squat	4	6	3min
5	3-point physioball push-ups	4	6	3min
6	Suspended Ring/TRX Inverted Rows	4	6	3min
7	KB/DB Ground to Upright Row	4	6	3min

Workout 4

Running intervals in kit.

Convert your best recent 5-mile time to seconds, divide it by 10, and now you have your 800 meter split time. Subtract at least 5 seconds from this time and use this for each 800 meter sprint time to complete.

- Run 6, 800m sprints
- Take 45 seconds of rest after each sprint.

After you've run the 6 sprints, find a level spot of ground that doesn't have any holes or bumps around it. Position your feet about shoulder-width apart and perform 3 sets of 8 maximal vertical jumps (yes, still in kit). Take 60 seconds of rest after each jump. These jumps should be separate and deliberate, not continuous.

Workout 5

	Exercise	Sets	Reps	Rest
1	Turkish Get-ups	1+4	6	2min
2	Weighted Rings/TRX Pull-ups	4	6	2min
3	Bulgarian SL Squat	4	6	2min
4	Ring/TRX suspended flyes	4	6	2min
5	Standing Cable/Hammer Row	4	6	2min
6	Wall/Hand-stand Push-ups	4	6	2min

Workout 6

- 4 rounds of Tailpipe (thanks to Gym Jones)
- bike for 45 minutes at 75-85% max heart rate (220-age x .75 and .85)
- 4 more rounds of Tailpipe

For Tailpipe:
- Hold 50-80 pounds of KBs or DBs (in semi-curl position with elbows almost on ribs)
- Row for 500 meters

Workout 7

	Exercise	Sets	Reps	Rest
1	DB Squat OH Press	4	12	60sec
1	DB Push-ups-Row-Row			
2	Walking weighted lunges	4	12	60sec
2	KB Swings			
3	Windmill Push-ups	4	12	60sec
3	Inverted plank rows			
4	Ring/TRX flyes	4	12	60sec

Note: Perform each same-numbered exercise as a part of a single super-set, rest for the indicated interval, then start the next set with the first exercise of the super-set; repeat to complete indicated number of sets.

Workout 8

- Run 3 miles with 40 pounds for best time
- After 3 minutes of rest following the run, perform the following complex:
-- Weighted Single-leg Backsquats (40 pounds)
-- Weighted chin-ups (40 pounds)
-- Weighted push-ups (40 pounds)

--- Perform the complex 6 times with 60 seconds rest between sets.
--- Perform 40 walking lunges per set and the maximum number of CONTROLLED and full range of motion repetitions for the chin-ups and push-ups that you can do.

Workout 9

After the RAW Movement Prep, do 5 minutes of jump rope at about 75% of your age-predicted max HR (220-age).
After that, a complex:
- Overhead squats
- Inverted rows

- Jammer

First do one warm-up set of 6 reps on each exercise. Next do a 1-->6 ladder with this complex, allowing one guy to go through the complex before the next guy starts.
Do 3 work sets of the complex (1-->6, 3 times), with no rest between the end of when you do the 6 reps of the complex and the 1 rep round of the complex.

Workout 10

	Exercise	Sets	Reps	Rest
1	Overhead Squat	3	8	60sec
2	KB Swings	3	8	60sec
2	Chin-ups			60sec
3	Dive-bomber push-ups	3	8	60sec
4	KB Squat to Press	3	8	60sec
6	Dynamax Ball Slams	3	8	60sec
6	Walking Lunges			

Note: Perform each same-numbered exercise as a part of a single super-set, rest for the indicated interval, then start the next set with the first exercise of the super-set; repeat to complete indicated number of sets.

RAW 2-week No Gym Workouts

- RAW Movement Prep prior to all workouts
- RAW Mobility/Flexibility drills after all workouts
- Recommended workout days: MON, TUES, WED, FRI, SAT
- Recommended rest days: THURS, SUN
  - Note: Rest = no workout at all

Workout 1

	Exercise	Sets	Reps	Rest
1	Wall Squat	5	5	30sec
2	Armor + Weight Pull-up	4	8	60sec
3	Ruck Squat	4	8	60sec
4	One-arm Push-up	4	5	60sec
5	Kit + Ruck lunges	4	8	60sec
6	Half-bent ruck row	4	8	60sec
7	Ruck L-Push-up	4	8	60sec

Workout 2

- Take your 5 mile run time and convert it to seconds
- Divide that by 10 and then subtract 15 seconds
- The number you get with the second bullet is your target time for each 800 meter sprint that you'll run, 10 times, with 60 seconds of rest in between each sprint.

Workout 3

	Exercise	Sets	Reps	Rest
1	Drop Jumps			
1	Weighted Jump to Pull-up	5	5	90sec
1	Crossover push-up to row			
2	Weighted step-ups			
2	Side block push-ups	4	5	60sec
2	Ruck Thrusters			
2	Upright Rows			

Note: Perform each same-numbered exercise as a part of a single complex, rest for the indicated interval, then start the next set with the first exercise of the complex; repeat to complete indicated number of sets.

Workout 4

Running intervals in kit.

Convert your best recent 5-mile time to seconds, divide it by 10, and now you have your 800 meter split time. Subtract at least 5 seconds from this time and use this for each 800 meter sprint time to complete.
- Run 6, 800m sprints
- Take 45 seconds of rest after each sprint.

After you've run the 6 sprints, find a level spot of ground that doesn't have any holes or bumps around it. Position your feet about shoulder-width apart and perform 3 sets of 8 maximal vertical jumps (yes, still in kit). Take 60 seconds of rest after each jump. These jumps should be separate and deliberate, not continuous.

Workout 5

	Exercise	Sets	Reps	Rest
1	Wall Squat	5	5	30sec
2	One arm Pull-ups	4	5	90sec
3	Heavy Ruck Carry	3	2min	60sec
4	Overhead Ruck Squat	4	12	60sec
5	Ruck Rows	4	12	60sec
6	Knee to Elbow Push-ups	4	12	60sec
7	Overhead Ruck Press	4	12	60sec

Workout 6

10 Rounds of the following:
- Farmer's Carry (use 2 rucks filled with 30-40 lbs each) for 100 meters
- Burpees (a.k.a. Squat Thrust) with no jump x 10 (increase to 12/15 when you can complete each set of 10)

Workout 7

	Exercise	Sets	Reps	Rest
1	Drop Jumps			
1	Weighted Jump to Pull-up	4	1→6	3min
1	Crossover push-up to row			
2	Weighted step-ups			
2	Side block push-ups	3	1→6	N/A
2	Ruck Thrusters			
2	Upright Rows			

Note: Perform each same-numbered complex of exercises in an upward ladder. This is best performed with 4-6 guys so that you each perform the iteration of reps and rotate out of the exercise. After you reach the 6 reps in a set, the next set begins with 1 rep.

Workout 8

- Run 3 miles with 40 pounds for best time
- After 3 minutes of rest following the run, perform the following complex:
-- Weighted Single-leg Backsquats (40 pounds)
-- Weighted chin-ups (40 pounds)
-- Weighted push-ups (40 pounds)

--- Perform the complex 6 times with 60 seconds rest between sets.
--- Perform 40 walking lunges per set and the maximum number of CONTROLLED and full range of motion repetitions for the chin-ups and push-ups that you can do.

Workout 9

- 5 minutes of jump rope (or small/mini hops/jumps if you don't have a rope) at about 75% of your age-predicted max HR (220-age).

After that, perform this complex:
- Overhead ruck squats
- Quick push-ups
- Upright ruck rows

First do one warm-up set of 6 reps on each exercise. Next do a 1→6 ladder with this complex, allowing one guy to go through the complex before the next guy starts.

Do 3 work sets of the complex (1-->6, 3 times), with no rest between the end of when you do the 6 reps of the complex and the 1 rep round of the complex.

Workout 10

	Exercise	Sets	Reps	Rest
1	Wall Squat	5	5	30sec
2	Armor + Weight Pull-up	4	8	60sec
2	Ruck Squat			
3	One-arm Push-up	4	5	60sec
4	Kit + Ruck lunges	4	8	60sec
4	Half-bent ruck row			
5	Ruck L-Push-up	4	8	60sec

Note: Perform each same-numbered exercise as a part of a single super-set, rest for the indicated interval, then start the next set with the first exercise of the super-set.

Nutrition

The meal plans provided below are only examples of the caloric intakes indicated. Specific individual dietary needs were not taken into consideration in preparation of these sample meal plans. Therefore, the meal plan examples are intended only as general caloric guidance, rather than a strict template to be followed exactly.

Meal/ Event	Foods	Amount	Calories	
3,000 kcal Diet for 1 day				
Early-morning snack	Toast whole wheat	1 slice	69	
	Jam	1tsp	17	
	Orange Juice	4oz	55	Total:141
AM workout	Sport Drink	12oz	90	
Breakfast	Orange Juice	4oz	55	
	Strawberries	1 cup	53	
	Egg hard cooked	1	78	
	Bran Cereal	1.5 cups	184	
	Milk 1%	8oz	110	
	Toast	1 slice	69	
	Margarine	1 tsp	34	
	Jam	1 tsp	17	
Midmorning snack	Bagel whole wheat	1 medium	320	
	Margarine	1 tsp	34	
	Jam	2 tsp	33	
	Coffee or tea	1 cup	0	
Lunch	Turkey sandwich			
	Turkey sliced	4oz	126	
	Bread whole wheat	2 slices	138	
	Mayo	2 tsp	70	
	Lettuce	1 leaf	0	
	Tomato	2 slices	8	
	Baked Lays	Bag	120	
	Apple	1 medium	80	
	Juice	8oz	144	Total:686
Afternoon snack	String cheese	1oz	80	
	Pretzels	1oz	108	
	Grapes	1 cup	60	Total: 248
Snack/2	Apple	1	90	
Dinner	Chicken vegetable stir-fry.			
	Chicken Breast	4oz	170	
	Broccoli	1 cup	44	
	Red pepper, carrots, celery, bean sprouts.	¼ cup each	59	
	Vegetable oil	2tsp	80	
	Soy sauce	To taste		
	Rice	2/3 cup cooked	137	
	Orange	1 medium	62	
	Tea	1 cup	0	Total:552
Evening snack	Milk 1%	8oz	100	
	Graham crackers	5 squares	75	Total:175
			Total calories: 2,979 Carb:483 grams Protein:139 grams Fat:64 grams Dietary fiber grams: 44	

4,000 Kcal Diet for 1-day			
Meal/ Event	Foods	Amount	Calories
Breakfast	Orange Juice	12oz	180
	Honeydew melon	¼ melon	115
	Cereal	2 cups	320
	Milk(1%)	1.5 cups	165
	Toast(whole wheat)	3 slice	210
	Margarine	2tsp	70
	Jam	1tsp	17
			Total: 1,077
Midmorning snack	Bagel(whole wheat)	1 medium	320
	Margarine	1tsp	35
	Jam	2tsp	35
	Coffee	1 cup	0
	Sport drink	18oz	135
			Total: 525
Lunch	Hamburger	3oz	215
	Hamburger roll	1 roll	230
	Ketchup	2tsp	10
	Lettuce	1 leaf	0
	Tomato	2 slices	12
	Potato wedges	½ cup	290
	Banana	1 medium	100
	V-8 Juice cocktail	8oz	50
			Total: 907
Afternoon snack	String cheese	1oz	115
	Saltine crackers	6 small	80
	Grapes	1 cup	60
	Sport drink	18oz	135
			Total: 390
Workout	Sport Drink	18oz	135
Dinner	Broiled salmon filet	4oz	185
	Broccoli	2 cups	90
	Margarine	2 tsp	70
	Baked potato	1 medium	190
	Sour cream	1 tbsp	30
	Fruit cocktail	1 cup fresh	120
			Total:685
Evening snack	Milk(1%)	1 cup	110
	Popcorn	3 cups microwaved	92
			Total:202
			Totals: 3,921 calories Carbs: 647 grams Protein: 145 grams Fat: 99 grams

Printed in Great Britain
by Amazon.co.uk, Ltd.,
Marston Gate.